This thing called
Sex

To Babbsy.
My love. My light.
My inspiration.

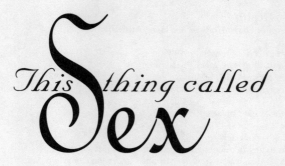

This thing called Sex

How to put more love, intimacy and sensuality into your life

Ian Oshlack

Illustrations by Robert Langley

HarperHealth
An imprint of HarperCollins*Publishers*

HarperHealth

An imprint of HarperCollins*Publishers*, Australia

First published in Australia in 1996
by HarperCollins*Publishers* Pty Limited
ACN 009 913 517
A member of the HarperCollins*Publishers* (Australia) Pty Limited Group

HarperCollins*Publishers*

25 Ryde Road, Pymble, Sydney NSW 2073, Australia
31 View Road, Glenfield, Auckland 10, New Zealand
77–85 Fulham Palace Road, London W6 8JB, United Kingdom
Hazelton Lanes, 55 Avenue Road, Suite 2900, Toronto, Ontario, M5R 3L2
and 1995 Markham Road, Scarborough, Ontario M1B 5M8, Canada
10 East 53rd Street, New York NY 10032, USA

The National Library of Australia Cataloguing-in-Publication data:

Oshlack, Ian.
    This thing called sex : how to put more love, intimacy and
    sensuality into your life.

    ISBN 0 7322 5673 9.

    1. Sex instruction. 2. Sensuality. I. Title
613.96

Designed by William Hung
Cover design by William Hung
Cover and text illustrations by Robert Langley
Typeset in Australia by Emtype Desktop Publishing
Printed in Australia by Griffin Paperbacks

9 8 7 6 5 4 3 2 1
99 98 97 96

Our thanks go to those who have given us permission to reproduce
copyright material in this book. Particular sources of print material
are acknowledged in the text. Every effort has been made to contact
the copyright holders of print material, and the publisher welcomes
communication from any copyright holder from whom permission
was inadvertently not gained.

Quotes by Osho Rajneesh on pages 11 and 135 reproduced with permission,
© Osho International Foundation.

Source of poem by Harriet L. Childe-Pemberton on page 140 is unknown.

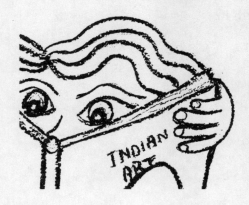

CONTENTS

NAMASTE

IN the Hindu tradition, namaste relates to the placing of one's palms together, bringing them to your face and bowing to another.

It means 'I give of myself, to you, in heartfelt thanks.'

Namaste is something you share with your beloved, prior to making love.

In the tradition of namaste, I give thanks to the following people, without whom this book would never have made it into existence.

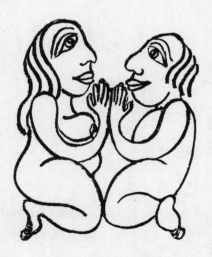

I would like to thank those people who, in one way or another, have been catalysts in my spiritual growth over the years: Stuart Wilde, Alan Lowen, Penny Cooke, David Ward, Janne Martinengo, Smito, Nityama and Stephan Kahlert.

Thanks are also due to the following people …

To Brenda Sutherland who had the first crack at the book when it was still in a form best described as embryonic and who gave her seal of approval on the final draft.

To Ann Holland, who read it and read it and read it and whose love and support throughout this project and beyond I will always cherish.

To Amalia Camateros, Cathy Hereen, Sandhi Spiers, Cynthia Connop, 'Fabulous' Phil Lukies, Robert Rice, Georgie Wain, Azurra and Yashu who provided continual encouragement, input and assistance, allowing me the confidence to maintain my direction.

To Robert Langley for going above and beyond the call of duty in providing the illustrations.

And finally to Osho. Wherever you are.

HOW TO
USE THIS BOOK

THE aim of this book is to enable you to create and maintain the erotic mystery that makes sex such a pleasurable experience.

At the same time it seeks to demystify sexuality, allowing you to view it from a new perspective.

Although you may find this book hard to put down, it is actually a book to be experienced, rather than read.

Either alone or with your partner.

If you are sharing this book with a partner, it is best that you take it in turns to read a chapter to each other. While one reads, the other lies in a comfortable position with their eyes closed.

As you try some of the exercises in this book, always remember that you only need to go as far as you feel comfortable. In so doing, it is vitally important that you communicate with your beloved which areas make you feel sensitive or excited or loving or inspired or whatever.

The more risk you take, the more you lower your boundaries, the more benefit you will receive.

Above all, have fun.

For this is what sex is all about.

> 'WHAT USE IS A BOOK,'
> THOUGHT ALICE, 'WITHOUT
> PICTURES OR CONVERSATIONS.'
>   Lewis Carroll

Sex:
How safe is it?

Because it looks at sex beyond penetration, much of what is in this book is as safe as it gets.

The level of risk inherent when partaking of any type of intimate activity with another person is in direct relation to your level of involvement; a one-night stand as distinct from a long-term committed relationship.

If you and your partner have been together for a short time, then when it comes to genital contact, it would be advisable for you to use a condom. While the risk involved in oral genital contact is not quite as pronounced, it would be prudent to refrain from this activity until your relationship has had a chance to evolve and/or you have both taken a blood test.

Taking an HIV test in today's sexual climate is quite a reasonable request of each other. Remember, to be absolutely sure you need to take the test twice, three months apart and at

> 'If you want to have sex, you've got to trust, at the core of your heart, the other creature.'
>
> D. H. Lawrence

the same time, being trusting of each other.

If you are in a long-term, committed and loving relationship then the need for protection (other than to prevent conception), is really not necessary.

Allow your common sense to prevail by following the guidelines in this book. You will find that when it comes to sex, you have nothing to fear except fear itself.

SEX BEYOND INTERCOURSE

This thing called sex is not intended to be a dissertation on the pros and cons of celibacy.

Or penetration.

Or sexual positions.

Or performance.

Simply put, this book is about intimacy.

And sensuality.

And touching.

And nurturing.

And caressing.

And kissing.

And stroking.

And pampering.

And hugging.

And fondling.

And squeezing.

And sucking.

And cuddling.

And caring.

And embracing.

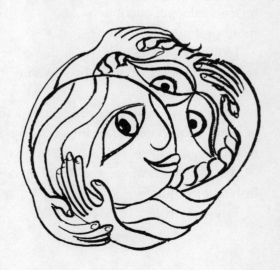

And holding.

And feeling.

And loving.

And orgasm.

Yes, orgasm.

At its most intense.

At its most profound.

At its most spiritual.

Whether you're a man or a woman.

It is also a book about change. And about knowing your boundaries and moving through them.

It is a book about honesty.

And trust.

And taking risks.

It is about exploring your untapped sexual potential and enhancing your loveplay. And finding love on a deeper and much more profound level.

> 'TODAY THE EMPHASIS IS ON SEX AND VERY LITTLE ON THE BEAUTY OF SEXUAL RELATIONSHIP.'
> Henry Miller

However, while this book looks at the intimate and sensuous aspects of sexuality, its aim is not to discourage intercourse.

Rather, you will discover that if and when intercourse occurs, it becomes the climax to an incredibly big and beautiful adventure.

An adventure where the act of making love lasts hours, instead of minutes.

Enjoy the ride.

THIS THING CALLED SEX

It is the most misunderstood of human foibles.

It is, therefore it isn't.

But what is it, really?

This most strange and exquisite of rituals.

This thing called sex.

This feeling of sexy.

This attitude that is sexual.

This enigma known as sexuality.

What is the key motivator, the trigger that unleashes the wave of passion?

The spirit of desire?

The surge of emotion?

The essence of sex?

Or is there a trigger at all?

Do we continually lock away our true feelings because of fear, guilt and shame?

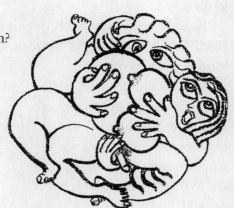

Even with our so-called enlightened civilisation, attitudes perpetrated by religion, community and family have created a society in which sex and sexuality are still very much repressed. They are

> 'SHAME IS THE FEELING YOU HAVE WHEN YOU AGREE WITH THE WOMAN WHO LOVES YOU THAT YOU ARE THE MAN SHE THINKS YOU ARE.'
>
> Carl Sandburg

still spoken of in hushed tones, with a hint of a snigger and a touch of embarrassment.

As a result of this repression, sex has become a topic that is discussed, analysed, scrutinised and exploited. Yet there is virtually no discussion that is open and rational. And nobody ever mentions intimacy and sensuality.

So, why is it that sex sells?

Why? Because it is the forbidden fruit. It's what we all want and desire but are afraid to grasp.

For many of us, sex can be the fine line between pleasure and pain.

Sex can make the strong weak and the weak strong.

Sex is a power that, in its own ethereal way, rules the planet.

Sex, above all, can elicit the most exquisite of emotions. It will satisfy the greatest hunger and restore the spirit of the most depressed of souls.

Sex is the lifeline to creativity. It captures our senses and enhances our existence. Without sex we would never know how to fly. With it, we can reach the stars.

> 'THE REDUCTION OF THE UNIVERSE TO A SINGLE BEING.'
>
> Victor Hugo

This, then, is a journey into your sexuality.

Your consciousness.

Your innocence.

A journey that will exhilarate you with its potential and inspire you with its wisdom.

It is an exploration that will take you to the multiplicity of emotional, creative and spiritual levels that sex has the ability to offer.

In this, the discovery of the true nature and dimension that constitutes sex, you will come to the realisation that when you reach the end, you will only be at the beginning.

THE MORE YOU CHANGE, THE BETTER YOU'LL FEEL

It has been said many times that change is, in fact, inevitable. For most of us, this is true.

And one of the most significant ways we encounter change is in our sexuality.

For as we grow, we learn.

As we mature, we understand.

As we explore, we experience.

This is the very nature of change.

However, when it comes to change in any part of our lives, we tend to do it reluctantly or resist it completely.

For change usually means altering the way we perceive our sexuality and the way we interact with our partner.

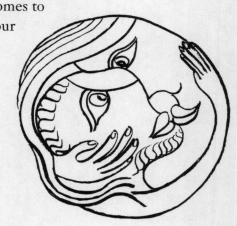

To get the most out of any relationship we have to be prepared to change, and in so doing overcome the fear of change by allowing it to happen. It

> 'THE MORE THINGS CHANGE, THE MORE THEY STAY THE SAME.'
>
> Alphonse Karr

will be in allowing change to happen that we will ultimately enhance the quality of our life and the quality of our lovemaking.

Many of us run away from change, especially where sex is involved. We would rather take what could be regarded as a transient, feel-good course of action.

The alternative is a kind of commitment.

In other words, you could follow the precepts of this book as singular exercises. In so doing you will find they will work either by opening your eyes to new horizons or by creating pleasurable experiences that last for a short time. When it's over, not much has changed.

Or you could take what this book reveals as a blueprint for change.

This does not mean altering your persona, but more changing your perceptions.

In the way you react and respond to yourself and your beloved.

In the way you act.

In the way you touch.

In the way you feel.

Think about your life at present. Are you living in a state of completeness? Are you experiencing bliss and ecstasy? Is there honesty in your relationships? When you make love, are you in love?

If the answer to any of these or any similar questions relating to your current state of being is no, then you probably need a shift in energy.

This shift does not have to be totally dramatic. But it does have to be total.

And in this totality lies the concept behind this book.

A concept for change.

For change *is* inevitable. Especially if you are to find the real joy that constitutes intimacy. But in order to find the intimate connection, you must first find yourself.

It is this that requires change.

If you choose to stay as you are – and as you are is the very thing that is holding you back – then it will become far more difficult to experience true intimacy.

For out of intimacy comes ecstasy. And ecstasy is the ultimate outcome of change.

Extraordinary things happen when you change.

Extraordinary things happen to you and to those around you.

You feel.

They feel.

Your passion.

Your energy.

Your love.

Your change.

From the past to the present.

From the present to the present.

And out of the present emerges something that is very special.

But the most extraordinary thing you'll discover when you change is that it is all so very ordinary. It is the inability to change that is really extraordinary.

So, whatever happens when you read this book, accept it as part of your change.

It's good for the soul.

It's good for the world.

It's good for you.

> 'CHANGE IS NOT MADE
> WITHOUT INCONVENIENCE,
> EVEN FROM WORSE TO BETTER.'
> Richard Hooker

THE BREATH OF LIFE

THE first thing we do when we come into this life is to inhale.

The last thing we do before we finally take leave of our body is to exhale.

In between arrival and departure it is only the inhalation and exhalation of the breath that maintains our aliveness.

It is the breath that is the key factor in the way we are in any given situation.

For no matter what our state of being, we never stop breathing.

> 'THE SECRET OF LIFE IS BREATH.'
> Anais Nin

When we are sick, we breathe.

When we sleep, we breathe.

When we are at play, we breathe.

When we meditate, we breathe.

When we make love, we breathe.

In fact, each and every day we inhale and exhale an average of 23 000 times. But do we ever stop and actually think about our breath?

The breath is not only the primary ingredient for survival, it is the method by which we channel our energy, regenerate our cells and maintain our equilibrium. It is also the way we connect with our feelings. However, because of our emotional suppression, many of us only breathe at the minimum of our capacity.

It is a strange anomaly in the human psyche that when we become excited or stimulated or invigorated or aroused we either forget to breathe or breathe harder.

When it comes to any act of intimacy, the harnessing of our sensual energy is centred around the way we breathe.

Because breathing is something we take for granted, the vast majority of us rarely get to experience the fullness of our breathing.

So, in order to get the most out of our sexuality, we must first discover the importance of breath and by becoming aware of our breathing, we can enhance the erotic experience.

We talk about the breath a lot throughout this book, as breathing is interconnected with many of the ways in which we can enhance, explore and focus on our sensuality.

And breathing is all about focus.

In yoga you breathe in and out through the nose, taking the breath through your chest to way down into your belly. You can actually feel the breath coming into your body and nurturing it. On the exhalation, the body lets go and relaxes.

> 'BREATH IS THE BRIDGE FROM THE BODY TO THE SOUL, FROM THE BODY TO THE MIND. IF YOU CAN REGULATE BREATHING — YOU HAVE POWER OVER YOUR MIND.'
>
> Osho Rajneesh

In terms of your sexuality, breathing is more likely to be done through the mouth.

Because the breath is the carrier of energy throughout the body, it is one of the most important components of sex.

To exemplify this, here is an exercise you can try.

✳ Lie down on your back on the floor, with your knees bent and together.

Your arms should be outstretched, with the palms facing downward.

On the inhalation, spread your knees apart, lift your hips and pelvis upward, turn the palms upward and let your eyes look behind you. Feel the breath come into your body, deep down into your belly.

Keep this position while holding the breath in.

Upon exhalation, allow your body to let go, relaxing into the original position.

Repeat this exercise ten to fifteen times.

On the last repetition, close your eyes and straighten your legs, feeling your body sink into the floor.

Lie in this position for as long as you like, feeling the breath enter and exit your entire body. Allow your thoughts to drift by like clouds.

Once you get into the rhythm of using your breath, you'll begin to understand how breathing in the context of love and intimacy becomes a conduit for your internal energy.

The more you breathe, the more you will create an entirely new level of sexual excitement.

Throughout this book there are many exercises, most of which involve breathing.

Now, take a deep breath and turn the page.

'TO INHALE THE DIVINE SPIRIT IS TO REGENERATE, TO PRODUCE; TO EXHALE THE DIVINE BREATH IS TO BREED AND NOURISH THE MIND.'

Bettina von Arnim

OVERCOMING GUILT

FOR many of us, when it comes to expressing and exploring our sexuality, we often come face to face with the feeling known as guilt. That what we are doing or thinking or saying or feeling is somehow wrong.

> 'IS SEX DIRTY?
> ONLY WHEN IT IS BEING
> DONE RIGHT.'
> Woody Allen

Or improper.

Or dirty.

Or even dishonourable.

Or it may be something we ought not to be doing, because we are afraid someone will find out.

Because it may be morally wrong.

And even though we find it enjoyable, why is it that we often experience feelings of guilt when it comes to sex?

Why does guilt enter our mind when we seek to learn more about our sexuality?

The answer lies in the emotion that constitutes guilt. An emotion that is usually the manifestation of the opinions, judgements and morals of others.

Guilt is all the 'shoulds' we have taken on over the years. 'You should do this.' 'You shouldn't do that.'

Whether it comes from our community, the church, society in general or our peers, the fear of sexuality that affects many individuals is translated into blinkered attitudes. It is not necessarily the narrow thinking of these people that creates

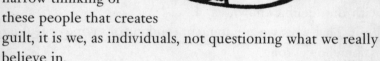

guilt, it is we, as individuals, not questioning what we really believe in.

We are all entitled to think, read and discuss whatever subject is of interest to us.

It is the transferring of our beliefs onto others and vice versa that is the root cause of feelings of guilt. And this is a major burden that we take with us from our childhood.

As children we were continually bombarded by the belief systems of our parents, teachers, religious leaders and friends.

However intentional or unintentional these senti-

> 'A MAN WHO HAS NOT PASSED THROUGH THE INFERNO OF HIS PASSIONS HAS NEVER OVERCOME THEM.'
>
> Carl Jung

ments were, they had a tendency to cover a wide range of topics in our lives. From sport to politics, to career, to spiritual and emotional issues. The opinions of others also affected our perceptions of morality and how we came to see ourselves as sexual beings.

It is these belief patterns that often manifest themselves in later life as feelings of shame.

And out of shame comes the feeling of guilt.

Guilt is an uncompromising emotion.

Because it is a product of the mind. It exists, and yet it doesn't.

For guilt and shame are triggered by fear.

That feeling you get when you are doing something you believe you are not supposed or allowed to be doing.

> 'FEAR BORN OF IGNORANCE IS WORSE THAN FEAR BORN OF KNOWLEDGE.'
>
> Dr Charles Hill

In other words, it is the expression of a belief pattern that does not belong to you.

Only you can alleviate your feelings of guilt by taking responsibility for your actions.

What you have to realise is that in exploring your sexuality and sensuality there is no reason to feel in the slightest bit guilty.

You can say, do, act or be anything, or anyone, simply by being yourself.

Without guilt.

Without shame.

Without fear.

If it has been said once, it's been said a thousand times,

'You have nothing to fear except fear itself.'

Once you take the step to do whatever pleases you, then the feeling of guilt simply dissipates.

There is no reprisal.

No recrimination.

Guilt simply ceases to exist.

Because it never really existed in the first place.

> 'THE GREAT PLEASURE IN LIFE
> IS DOING WHAT PEOPLE SAY
> YOU CANNOT DO.'
>
> Walter Bagehot

LOVING YOURSELF

BEFORE you can give love, you must feel love.

Before you can make love, you must experience love.

Before you can talk of love, you must be in love.

And the first and most important love of your life is you. The lover within.

For in finding the lover within, you will be finding yourself.

And finding yourself will lead to loving yourself.

It is in the state of loving yourself that you'll be able to share your love with another.

For when it comes to self-love, the problem we all face at some time during our lives is the way society dictates how and what we should be.

That image of so-called perfection that none of us can live up to, because it is false.

For it is underneath the facade that true beauty really lies, and by bringing it to the surface it has a transformational effect.

However, allowing ourselves to make this discovery can be difficult.

The assumption that what we are is not what others want us to be is a total misconception.

It is this that leads us into creating an image of ourselves that does not equate with reality.

Our body shape.

Our face.

Our stomach.

Our hair.

Our wrinkles.

Our stretch marks.

Our scars.

And so on.

> 'A WOMAN IS TRULY BEAUTIFUL ONLY WHEN SHE IS NAKED AND SHE KNOWS IT.'
>
> Andre Courreges

The truth in all of this is that in the eyes of your lover, all of these aspects are objects of great beauty and desire. They are distinctive to you and are what makes you a unique individual.

But first you have to learn to accept and embrace them.

To love all of those parts of your body that make up the whole.

Because, once you learn to love and accept yourself, then the loving of another becomes an easier, richer and more meaningful experience.

Stand clothed, in front of a mirror, preferably a full-length mirror.

Look at yourself.

Observe the way you are and name all those things about you that you like. And all those parts that you may feel uncomfortable with.

Once you have done that for a short while, look yourself in the eyes and begin to observe your feelings.

What you think about yourself.

How you could learn to love yourself.

All the stuff that's going on inside you.

As you are doing this, keep breathing deeply.

Now slowly get undressed in front of the mirror. Observe yourself as you take off pieces of clothing. As parts of your body become exposed.

Your arms.

Your legs.

Your buttocks.

Your belly.

Your breasts.

Your genitals.

Stand there and look at yourself naked. And keep breathing.

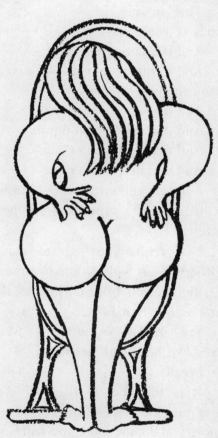

Look at yourself breathing.

As before, observe yourself from every aspect. Let your eyes stay on those areas that you don't really like and start to see the positive side of them.

After you have scanned your entire body, look deeply into your eyes.

Hold the gaze.

Breathing into the feeling.

And realise that you are not your body, but in your body.

> 'SOMETIMES THIS FACE LOOKS SO FUNNY,
> THAT I HIDE BEHIND A BOOK,
> SOMETIMES THIS FACE HAS SO MUCH CLASS,
> THAT I SNEAK A SECOND LOOK.'
> Phoebe Snow

That in this body is where you live.

And it is beautiful.

And in this acceptance of yourself, tell yourself what an exquisite butt you have.

And those great legs.

And that sensational figure.

And that sensuous mouth.

And that delectable nose.

And that cute little belly-button.

Concentrate especially on those bits you felt weren't attractive.

Now return your gaze to your eyes for a few minutes. Observe your feelings and breathe into them.

By now you'll begin to realise that you are a very special and unique human being.

See yourself as the incredibly beautiful person you really are.

> 'MAN IS HARDER THAN A
> ROCK AND MORE FRAGILE
> THAN AN EGG.'
> Yugoslav proverb

It is this feeling that you must cultivate. For the more you do, the more you will begin to believe in yourself.

Finish the process by continuing to look deep within your eyes and say to yourself, 'I feel a great love within my heart for you.'

Go up close to the mirror and kiss yourself.

Take a step back, close your eyes and take in three deep breaths.

As you inhale, feel your new-found love and vibrancy.

As you exhale, let go of all those negative feelings you had about yourself.

Let go of all those adverse opinions.

Let go of your ego, for the ego has no place in your life.

You are what you are and you accept all things.

The most important aspect about this process is that it is the first and last time you do it in front of a mirror, for the mirror is only a tool to your self-awareness.

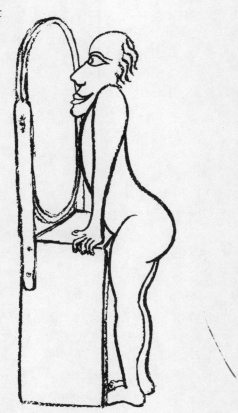

After all, what you see in the mirror is merely a reflection. Observing it is fine in the context of finding yourself. But now it is no longer necessary, for you have discovered your inner beauty and this is not what you see in the mirror.

You have passed through the form.

Of course, there will be occasions when feelings of self-doubt may creep back. It is at these times that you may need to reaffirm your power by simply repeating this mantra to yourself, 'I am what I am. And I am beautiful.'.

Say it with real conviction and meaning.

Say it because you believe it.

Say it with a genuine love for yourself.

You are what you are.

And you are beautiful.

> 'LOVE IS, ABOVE ALL,
> A GIFT OF ONESELF.'
> Jean Anoulth

JUDGING A BOOK
BY ITS COVER

THROUGHOUT our lives, as we connect and disconnect with people, the way we perceive each other is an important component in the way we relate.

And more often than not, what we see is not what we get.

How many times, when we're part of a gathering, where some of the people are strangers, do we look at someone and form an opinion about what they are, what they're like and their potential as sexual partners?

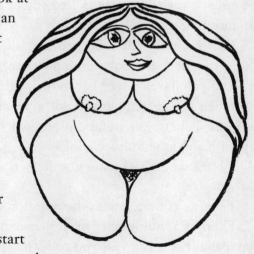

Moreover, the instant we make a decision to approach a stranger our relationship to them changes. We start to question ourselves and create scenarios about what to say, how we will say it, whether or not they will accept us or reject us, and so on.

For many of us, actually making eye contact with another person elicits fear. We turn away, afraid to look back.

These are some of the mind games we play when we seek to make a connection with another person. The reality of these games is that they are all a lie.

> 'SEX AND BEAUTY ARE ONE THING, LIKE FLAME AND FIRE. IF YOU HATE SEX, YOU HATE BEAUTY. IF YOU LOVE LIVING BEAUTY, YOU HAVE A REVERENCE FOR SEX.'
>
> D. H. Lawrence

Think about it.

Once you get to know a little about a stranger, how often are you 'right' in your perceptions?

Because our initial contact with another person is visual, we receive only a glimpse of their inner reality.

Their voice may carry a certain timbre.

The way they feel and respond when you touch them, whether it is shaking hands, hugging or kissing them, opens up differing realities.

The more intimate you become, the more you will discover that they also have a unique taste and smell.

And you haven't even got to their mind!

When you include aspects of a person such as intellect, attitude, beliefs, humour, opinions and spirituality, you end up with a unique human being.

A human being who was not the person you first laid eyes on.

Then, of course, comes the question of sexuality.

There is a multiplicity of desires and taboos that people have about sex. But can you tell what these are from your initial contact?

The person with the movie star looks and the most perfectly tuned body could carry many an emotional or sexual hang-up, while the individual who is a little softer and rounder and not so flawless physically may well be a steaming volcano of desire.

> 'IF YOU LACK BEAUTY, YOU LIVE THIS BEAUTY OUT IN THE OTHER. BUT IT IS THE SAME WITH UGLINESS.'
>
> Anais Nin

Society today places much on the superficial. The way we dress, do our hair, our face, the way we walk and the way we act. All these aspects are aimed at making that first contact a lasting impression. But it is the deeper aspects of a person that makes them more meaningful.

As you discovered in the previous chapter, we are not our bodies alone. The reality is that our bodies are merely vehicles for carrying our true selves.

The body is only form. And when you explore beyond the form, it is then that you will discover the real person.

So it is unwise to judge a book by its cover.

Explore the first few chapters. If they appeal to your sensibilities, you may realise that this is the kind of story that you can't put down.

> 'MAN WILL BECOME BETTER ONLY WHEN YOU WILL MAKE HIM SEE WHAT HE IS LIKE.'
>
> Anton Chekhov

BEAUTY IS
IN THE EYES ...

'WELCOME,
I SAW YOU COMING FROM AFAR,
I SEE YOU NOW,
AND YOU ARE BEAUTIFUL.'

THESE words come from Africa's Kalahari Bushmen. When said with sincerity, they can have a profound impact.

When you come together with your beloved after being apart or as you sit together prior to making love, look into their eyes and with all the love you are feeling, whisper the verse to each other in turn.

When you come to the last line, 'And you are beautiful', keep repeating it several times, looking deeper and deeper into your beloved's eyes.

The deeper you go, the more you will become aware of an inner entity within your beloved that exists beyond the outer body.

When you look into the eyes of another, you not only see, but also feel.

It is in the eyes of your lover that aspects of their inner nature are revealed. As well as your own.

It is said that the eyes are the window to the soul. They are also a mirror to your own disposition.

For many, gazing into another person's eyes can elicit a sense of unease. We feel discomfort, as if our thoughts are being intruded on or that we are the intruder.

Intrusive as you may believe it to be, gazing into another's eyes reveals the frontiers across which information is transmitted, issues addressed and love crystallised.

But looking into another's eyes with a sense of affection can impart a series of totally different feelings.

Tenderness.

Passion.

Empathy.

Longing.

And trust.

What this means is that, except on rare occasions, it is best not to have an intimate encounter with the lights out.

> 'LOVE DOES NOT RECOGNISE THE DIFFERENCE BETWEEN PEASANT AND MIKADO.'
>
> Japanese proverb

For in the absence of light you can lose a certain level of intimacy.

The visuality of observing and watching the waves of pleasure.

Of seeing the changes in the colour and clarity of your beloved's skin, hair, feet, knees, navel, nose, ears, lips, genitals and eyes.

Eye contact will put a new connectedness back into the mutual pleasure you are giving to and receiving from each other.

As an exercise, sit facing each other.

Ideally you will do this on the floor or on a bed.

And you should be naked.

When you are in a comfortable position facing each other, close your eyes for a moment.

Gently inhale, imagining the breath being drawn in through your genitals.

Now exhale, allowing the breath out via your genitals.

As you breathe, you will feel a warm glow start to flow throughout your body.

You will also become aware of the close proximity of your loved one.

After a few minutes, without saying a word, take in a deep breath and, as you exhale, open your eyes and look into those of your beloved.

You will see a new image of your lover.

It will be like seeing each other for the first time.

A vibrancy and aliveness will have emerged as their inner beauty becomes apparent.

Let your eyes wander over your partner's face, hair, neck, body, arms, legs. Observe the way they are formed.

The curvature.

The nooks and crannies.

The blemishes.

The textures.

As you continue to observe your partner, feel their gaze upon you.

It is OK to feel a little discomfort or excitement or sadness or even foolishness.

You may feel that you want to cry or laugh or just be silent, observing the wonder of your beloved.

Be aware of the breath. Breathe in the other's presence.

Their energy.

Their warmth.

Their closeness.

Their love.

The fact that you are there together.

> 'WHY NOT BE ONESELF? THIS IS THE WHOLE SECRET OF SUCCESSFUL APPEARANCE ... IF ONE IS A GREYHOUND, WHY LOOK LIKE A PEKINESE?'
>
> Edith Sitwell

Two beings who have a deep and intense bond between each other.

A shared communion.

A profound love.

When you feel the time is right, whisper the mantra to each other.

Welcome,
I saw you coming from afar,
I see you now,
And you are beautiful
And you are beautiful
And you are beautiful
And you are so very beautiful.

Then putting your arms out, gently touch each other. Drawing yourselves together for a loving embrace. Holding each other, feeling the energy between you. Feeling the love.

For in this togetherness you will have discovered that beauty is, indeed, in the eye of the beholder.

Welcome.

> 'APPEARANCES, OFTEN,
> ARE DECEIVING.'
>
> Aesop

REJECTING REJECTION

LOOKING into your beloved's eyes (or anyone else's eyes for that matter) and saying 'You are beautiful' may sound like a simple process. But in many instances it is not as easy as it sounds.

Especially if the feeling is not reciprocated.

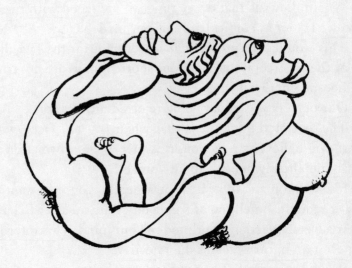

During our formative years, through adolescence and into adulthood, one of the main reasons we lose much of our self-esteem is because of rejection.

Rejection can come in a variety of forms:

Being criticised by another person.

Not being invited to a party or function.

Asking someone out on a date and being knocked back.

Or having a sexual request refused.

When incidents like this occur, it can be a truly painful experience. The more we are rejected, the more painful it becomes, and the more we tend to blame ourselves for being rejected.

This can lead to self-rejection, resulting in our lives becoming a reflection of our own internal self-doubt.

We think we're unworthy. That there is something wrong with the way we look or the way we are. Or that people just don't like us.

What follows is that every time we are faced with rejection we take it as confirmation of our inadequacy.

This would be a problem, if it were not for the fact that all of these perceptions about our shortcomings are not true.

Let me say that again.

Our perceptions about being rejected are not true.

The fact of the matter is that when you are faced with what you believe is rejection, it is merely an affirmation of what you already believe about yourself.

It's symptomatic of a situation whereby you may want to ask or request something of somebody, but you already have their adverse reaction imprinted in your mind. This internal expectation in turn creates the rejection.

If you are critical of someone, then what you see in them

is in reality a reflection of your own beliefs about yourself. This includes those judgements about what you imagine to be good and bad about the other person.

Conversely, if you believe every bit of criticism and rejection that is thrust upon you, then you will feel it. The pain. The agony. And the loss of self-esteem.

It will also create a lot of fear. And this fear is manifested from our inability to believe in ourselves as unique individuals.

This is why, for many of us, standing in front of a mirror elicits feelings of terror due to our self-perpetuating criticism.

Looking deep within ourselves is vastly different to looking at ourselves when we have a shave or put on our make-up. At these times what we see is superficial. It is the mask we wear in order to conform to what we believe to be society's accepted image of us. It is the mask we use to cover our inner emotional and sensual reality.

> 'IN ORDER TO BE REJECTED YOU MUST FIRST BE CONSIDERED.'
> Rev. Jesse Jackson

So by repeating the mirror process a number of times without the mirror, you will start to rid yourself of the apprehension you get when confronted by rejection. (The mirror process is described in the chapter 'Loving yourself'.)

You can even expand on this exercise by sitting quietly with a sheet of paper.

On one half of the paper write down all those reasons you feel rejected.

The thoughts and beliefs that are in opposition to the complete acceptance of 'I am beautiful'.

Once you start, do not stop writing.

No matter how silly it sounds, just keep scribbling.

Keep writing until there is nothing left.

Once you have finished, close your eyes for a moment.

Now read through what you have written.

Breathe into those feelings that may surface.

Now, on the other half of the sheet opposite the negative thoughts write down all those positive aspects about yourself.

When you have completed the list, read the positive thoughts out aloud.

Telling yourself how exquisitely beautiful you are. Because it is the truth.

Telling yourself what a wonderful and unique person you are. Because it is the truth.

Connect with your own personal power, allowing this energy to become you. Because it is the truth.

The longer you say the affirmations, the more intense will be the acceptance of yourself.

And the more you come to know and accept yourself the way you are, the more you will realise that rejection is a fallacy.

This is because you will now carry a resonance about you that, surprisingly, will cause people to react to you differently.

Self-doubt and self-rejection will become things of the past.

Old habits don't die so hard, after all.

> 'TO LOVE ONESELF IS THE BEGINNING OF A LIFE-LONG ROMANCE.'
>
> Oscar Wilde

PLEASURING
YOUR BODY

SELF-PLEASURING or masturbation, as some would call it, can be a highly erotic experience. Yet, for many people, the very act of touching some of the more intimate and sensitive parts of their own body can elicit strong feelings of guilt and shame.

Self-pleasure is a vital component of self-love and there is no reason why you cannot be at one with yourself. As such, guilt and shame are incompatible bedfellows with self-love.

> 'I'LL COME AND MAKE LOVE TO YOU AT FIVE O'CLOCK. IF I'M LATE, START WITHOUT ME.'
> Tallulah Bankhead

When it comes to self-love, your body is a veritable minefield of pleasure spots. And this loving of yourself is a wonderful way to heal any guilt and shame you may feel about your own sexuality.

If you're not too sure about what parts of your body constitute those areas of greatest sensitivity, here's a short exercise you may like to try.

Lie on your back on a bed, closing your eyes and taking deep breaths. On each exhalation allow yourself to sink into the mattress.

Run your fingers over
your body.

Stroke and caress
your nipples.

Your belly.

Your face.

Your hair.

Your inner
thighs.

Your genitals.

If there are parts
of your body you have
never touched in an erotic
manner before, now is the time
to take a little risk.

Become aware of any area that you may be apprehensive
about.

Focus your attention on it.

Slowly let your fingers creep closer to it.

Then, ever so lightly, stroke it. As you do, breathe into
any thoughts or feelings that come up.

Whatever you do, don't
back off. Just keep lightly
caressing the spot.

As you continue to ex-
plore your body, sooner or
later you are highly likely
to feel arousal in the area

> 'SHE WAS SOON MEDITATING
> AND MASTURBATING AND
> FINDING HERSELF DISSOLVED
> INTO THE COSMIC.'
> Alice Walker

of your genitals. This may be the result of direct contact or
the fact that you may be touching a particularly sensitive
part of your body.

It may well be something you are already aware of or it may be a new discovery. Whatever the reason, just lie back and enjoy the feeling.

The more you stroke and play with your body, the higher the state of excitement, the closer you will come to an orgasmic experience. It is at this point that feelings of self-doubt or sadness may surface. If they do, just keep breathing and ignore any adverse inclinations – simply ride the wave of pleasure.

As discussed in the chapter 'Ejaculation …', try to avoid actually releasing by breathing into the feeling. The aim of self-pleasuring is to get in touch with your erotic body. This will allow you to become more in tune with your orgasmic nature.

However, if you do get to a point where you can't hold the need for ejaculation any longer, then let it go and enjoy the explosion. When it happens, stay in touch with the breath. For in the aftermath of ejaculation there is a space for deep meditation. This is because ejaculation, when it occurs in the context of self-pleasuring, is not based on performance.

> 'MASTURBATION: THE PRIMARY SEXUAL ACTIVITY OF MANKIND. IN THE NINETEENTH CENTURY IT WAS A DISEASE; IN THE TWENTIETH IT IS A CURE.'
>
> Thomas Szasz

If it feels good, it is good.

Only you know your own body and exactly where you like to be touched.

And how you like to be touched.

And for how long you like to be touched.

The possibilities are endless. This is because touch knows no boundaries.

Once you become aware of the sensual potential of your body and are able to revel in it, then you'll be more able to give pleasure to another.

As you would to yourself.

'NO MAN IS A HYPOCRITE IN HIS PLEASURES.'

Samuel Johnson

WHAT'S LOVE GOT TO DO WITH IT?

EVERYTHING.

Or, it should be everything. However, if one is to believe the attitude that is prevalent in society today, sex and love are separate entities.

This is not to suggest that sex without love cannot be erotic.

It can be. Provided you play your cards right.

Such one-off dalliances are nearly always charged with a high level of emotion. Even so, because such a liaison constitutes sex on a different level, it needs to be placed into its true perspective.

For sex to be raised from the merely erotic to the blissfully ecstatic, you need love. This is because, in love, sex is sacred.

In love, sex is exploring and satisfying each other's desires.

In love, sex is experiencing each other's emotions.

> 'YOU MUST NOT FORCE SEX TO DO THE WORK OF LOVE OR LOVE TO DO THE WORK OF SEX.'
>
> Mary McCarthy

Consequently, sex in the context of love becomes an extension of that love. And because love is on a higher emotional plane than sex, it does not need to be sexual.

It is this increased level of awareness that transforms an act of sex into an act of love.

What's love got to do with it?

Everything.

A KISS IS
STILL A KISS

In its role as a shared experience, kissing is an act of individuality.

Your kiss is as unique as your fingerprint. The ultimate expression of the way you feel.

The way you are.
Your innermost potential.

Kissing is an intimate connection. Either as a preliminary exploration or as the aftermath of an ecstatic experience.

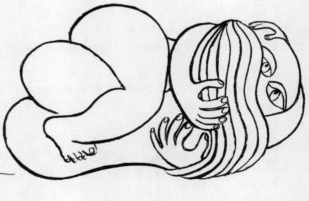

Kissing is the most personal aspect of sex. For in each kiss you give and receive a part of each other.

With each kiss, you become in touch with yourself and your beloved.

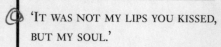

'IT WAS NOT MY LIPS YOU KISSED, BUT MY SOUL.'

Judy Garland

With each kiss, you and your beloved strike the same chord, in perfect harmony.

For when it comes to kissing, you are neither the kisser nor the kissed.

You become the kiss.

And the kiss need not have any ritual.

Need not have any time.

Need not have any place.

It can happen when it happens, whenever. Passionate, exciting, spontaneous, delicious, affectionate, tender and loving.

But remember, the most important kiss of all is the first.

And the last.

And all those in between.

Whether at the break of day or to say good night.

In greeting or parting.

Or as a prelude or epilogue to making love.

Kisses to savour.

Deeply.

Exploring.

Allowing.

To treat with all due reverence.

'YOU MUST REMEMBER THIS,
A KISS IS STILL A KISS,
A SIGH IS JUST A SIGH,
THE FUNDAMENTAL THINGS APPLY
AS TIME GOES BY.'

Herman Hupfeld

To give and receive at their quintessential moment.
When connection occurs and the time is conducive.
Which is why a kiss is still a kiss.

TO HUG AND BE HUGGED

HUGGING is the epitome of duality.

But in today's world, many believe it should be restricted to intimate situations.

While hugging is an important component of lovemaking, it need not be restricted to a singular time and place.

For hugging is inherent in our very nature.

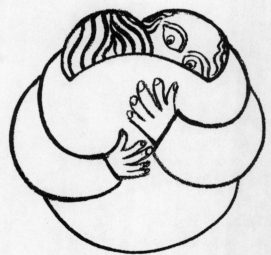

To envelop another person, of either sex, in a long, warm, lingering hug is to impart your innermost feelings for that person.

For hugs can say a lot about your warmth, your inhibitions, your demeanour. About you as a person.

A hug can happen anywhere, at any time.

For no reason at all.

Or with anyone.

Friends, associates or your beloved.

When you greet each other, hug.

In the morning, on arising, hug.

In the shower together, hug.

When you say goodbye to each other, hug.

And, of course, before and after you make love.

'TOO MUCH OF A GOOD THING CAN BE WONDERFUL.'

Mae West

To be affective, whether lying down or standing, a hug must be total and all encompassing. Your chest, belly, pelvis and legs need to be in contact with each other, arms firmly around the body.

And no back-slapping.

As you hold each other, be aware of your breathing, especially as you exhale, allowing your body to melt into the other. Becoming the hug.

Be aware of the other's energy.

Inhale their aroma.

Feel their affection.

For in the embrace of a hug you are enacting the most powerful and basic of needs.

The need to be held.

To be caressed.

To be squeezed.

For hugging is the unification of two beings in togetherness. The purest manifestation of love.

FINDING SANCTUARY

ONE of the ways to enhance your lovemaking is to alter the dynamics of where you normally do it. Ideally, this means setting up an area that becomes your spiritual place.

Your sanctuary.

A space that need not be permanent, but is created for the occasion.

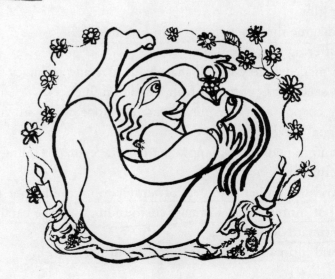

It may be a spare room or a part of your main living area.

Or you may simply wish to alter the ambience of your bedroom.

In many ways, it is best to set up this area at floor level, the centrepiece being a futon or thin mattress covered with silk, satin or whatever type of sheets you desire.

Use sarongs, shawls and other patterned materials to set the ambience.

Burn incense and intoxicating oils to enhance the atmosphere.

Surround the area with candles and flowers and soft toys and other things that are special to you and are an intrinsic part of your soul.

Let your creativity flow and the end result will be a space that exudes your combined sensuality.

Ensure you have your favourite music to play and plenty of iced water, fruits and other exotic edibles on hand.

Turn out the lights and just allow the candles to give off their glow.

Imagine the space has its own invisible walls.

Offering supreme privacy.

A place where you will share your love and intimacy.

A sanctuary, protected from outside influences.

A cocoon that surrounds and envelops you and your partner.

Your sanctuary will now start to take on a feeling of anticipation.

And the higher the level of anticipation, the higher the level of intimacy. For intimate surroundings are the catalyst of intimate occurrences.

And intimate occurrences lead to intimacy itself.

INITIATING INTIMACY

ONCE you have created your sanctuary, entering it and being a part of it requires a certain amount of ritual.

Whether or not you have created a special space or are just going to bed, this ceremony can be a wonderful initiation to many sessions in which you and your partner share your love.

It is a way of grounding each of you, by bringing you into the moment.

For this process allows you to connect with each other on both a physical and a spiritual level.

> 'RITUAL IS THE ORIGINAL WOMB OF ART. ITS WATERS CONTINUE TO NOURISH CREATIVITY.'
>
> Miriam Simos

To commence, play a piece of music that you both feel is appropriate to the occasion.

Stand clothed, but barefoot, facing your partner.

Observe each other's form in the warm glow of candles.

Now, close your eyes and inhale.

Smell the aromas and feel any subtle shifts in energy.

Be aware of the breath as it enters and exits your body.

Imagine it coming in through the top of your head and out through your heart.

Connect with your own inner feelings.

How those feelings integrate with your beloved.

How your beloved's presence is influencing the way you feel and the way you are.

Now open your eyes and gaze into the eyes of your partner.

Maintain this eye contact for a few minutes.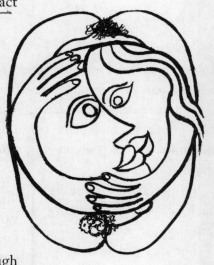

Breathing in your partner's energy.

Their presence.

Their beauty.

Their being.

Their love.

Without saying a word, each lightly cradle the other's face in one hand.

Stroke their cheek.

Run your fingers through their hair.

Look closely at each other.

Lightly kiss each other's face, ears, eyes, nose, neck, mouth.

Slowly allow yourselves to melt into a deep, all encompassing hug. As you do, be aware of any changes in the way you feel within yourself and about the person you are with.

When the time feels right, slowly separate, as you return to making eye contact.

It is now time to disrobe each other, taking it in turns to slowly and sensually remove one piece of clothing at a time. Undress your beloved as you, yourself, have always wanted to be undressed.

Remember, you must alternate. You remove an item of clothing from your beloved, then they reciprocate and so on.

> 'IF NOBODY HAD LEARNED TO UNDRESS, VERY FEW PEOPLE WOULD BE IN LOVE.'
> Dorothy Parker

As you discard a garment, stroke, caress and/or kiss that part of the other's body that becomes exposed.

Once you are both naked, give each other another lingering hug.

Allow your bodies to touch from top to bottom.

As each intertwines with the other, feel your collective energies unite.

You are one in the embrace.

Cheek to cheek.

Chest to chest.

Pelvis to pelvis.

Leg to leg.

Feel the warmth of their body, the softness of their skin, the gentleness of their touch.

> 'ONCE MORE I WILL SHYLY LET YOU UNDRESS ME AND GENTLY UNLOCK MY SEALED JEWEL.'
> Huang O

Inhale their aroma.

Run your hands down their back.

Squeeze their buttocks.

Run your fingers through their hair.

Closing your eyes, allow your lips to meet.
- Not kissing, but becoming the kiss.
- Becoming the passion.
- Becoming the love.

Creating the embryo of arousal.

The seed of seduction.

The source of surrender.

Now sit opposite gazing into each other's eyes.

Holding each other's hands.

Right palm facing down, left palm facing up.

As you breathe, imagine the inhalation entering through your left hand and the exhalation leaving through your right.

Be with this feeling as you continue looking deeply into each other's eyes.

The longer you are with your beloved in this way, the more you will perceive their inner glow.

The more you will feel their loving energy.

The more you will experience your unique connection.

How long you remain in this space is up to you. There will be times when you will want to sit in this manner for a long period. Or you may sit this way for only a few moments. There is no predetermined duration.

When the mood feels right, place your palms together as in a prayer position, bringing them to the front of your face, bowing forward as you touch foreheads.

Now say, in turn, to each other, 'I honour this sanctuary we have created and I honour you [name] as an aspect of myself.'

By completing this connection you have allowed your union to become integrated and, thus, you have laid the foundation for whatever it is that may happen to follow.

If anything.

For perfection may simply be the two of you together.

In each other's arms.

One with the other.

Or allowing the ambience of the space to create its own direction.

And as you will discover in the pages that follow, not only will that direction lead you to a virtually limitless variety of pleasurable pursuits, but these pursuits will now happen with more spirituality, more passion and more intimacy.

> 'LOVE SOUGHT IS GOOD, BUT
> GIVEN UNSOUGHT IS BETTER.'
>> William Shakespeare

ARE YOU GOOD IN BED?

WELL, are you?

If you answer in the affirmative then you are a better person than most.

Being 'good in bed' is an extremely subjective concept. Yet it is a concept that is not often questioned.

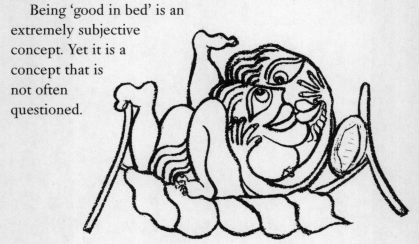

Just what does being 'good in bed' mean?

How important is it to know whether we are 'good in bed'?

And if we ask the question of someone, what answer do we expect?

Is our curiosity about how good someone is in bed really about having our own innermost desires satisfied?

And that being 'good in bed' is in reality the other person's willingness and ability to fulfil those desires?

In truth, the word 'good' does not enter the equation because we are all different sexually.

If intercourse is the main criterion of your loveplay, then 'good' may refer to how long the man can perform without ejaculating and whether or not the woman reaches any kind of climax.

> 'TWO SOULS WITH BUT A SINGLE THOUGHT,
> TWO HEARTS THAT BEAT AS ONE.'
>
> Maria Lovell

On the other hand, being 'good' may mean that either or both partners enjoy performing oral sex.

If you are both sensitive and caring and enjoy the languid sensuality that comes with true intimacy, then your sexual liaisons will last as long as you want. This can also be described as 'good'.

The way we react with one person will differ from the way we react with another. In some encounters, the chemistry may elevate the event to the very epitome of passion or may simply be soft and nurturing.

Ideally, you will be in connection with a partner who not only is open to expressing and sharing their emotions, but also has the desire to indulge in a wide cross-section of intimate experiences.

In other words, being good in bed is based on sexual and mutual compatibility.

You're only as good as each other.

Are you good in bed?

Yes, we are.

If you enjoy a high level of sexual enjoyment with another person, then the word 'good' becomes meaningless.

Because the pleasure you derive from each other 'just is'.

It just is.

And the more it is, the better it gets.

That's the real meaning of being good ... together.

> 'WHEN I'M GOOD, I'M VERY
> GOOD, BUT WHEN I'M BAD,
> I'M BETTER.'
>
> Mae West

THE FOREPLAY MYTH

BECAUSE there has been much sexual repression in Western society, our sex education has been somewhat lacking.

Most books on the subject emphasise sexual performance, rather than getting involved in discussing the giving and receiving of pleasure.

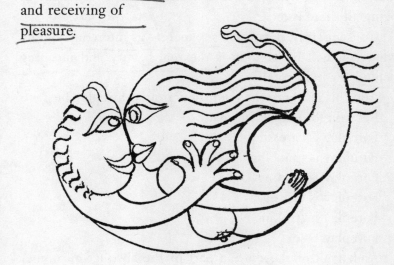

What most of us know about sex we either picked up from these manuals or learned from practical experience.

One question that may be floating around your head could be 'If this book is about sex beyond intercourse, what, then, is foreplay?'

> 'HER PASSIONS ARE MADE OF NOTHING BUT THE FINEST PART OF PURE LOVE.'
> William Shakespeare

Through our tentative early encounters, we discovered that one needed to indulge in an activity called foreplay, prior to penetration.

However, when one talks about foreplay, one needs to ask 'Foreplay to what?'

The common answer is 'Foreplay to sex', foreplay being regarded as a way of getting your partner 'turned on'.

As such, foreplay is seen as something separate from intercourse, which is still incorrectly perceived by many as being all there is to sex.

Consequently, if you see sex merely as intercourse, then what you will be missing is the real beauty and meaning behind sex in its totality.

And this is where the confusion around foreplay lies.

Because foreplay is intimacy.

Foreplay is caressing.

Foreplay is touching.

Foreplay is holding.

Foreplay is kissing.

Foreplay is stroking.

Foreplay *is* sex.

And if all of these are a part of the abstract misnomer 'foreplay', then foreplay, by implication, does not exist. It becomes merely a prelude to intercourse that deprives us of our spontaneity.

When you're with your beloved be patient, gentle and caring rather than going for the big bang. In so doing, you will be able to prolong your sexual encounter for as long as you desire.

What all this means is that intercourse becomes much more integrated into your entire sexual relationship.

When you and your beloved are together in intimacy, it should be viewed for what it is.

Not as a precursor for something else.

For that something else is only a myth.

> 'PLEASURE WITHOUT JOY IS AS HOLLOW AS PASSION WITHOUT TENDERNESS.'
>
> Alan Jay Lerner

THE IMPERCEPTIBILITY
OF TOGETHERNESS

WHEN you and your partner come together in union, you will notice physiological changes in each other.

Change that occurs as arousal takes hold and sensuality is heightened.

Change in our facial and bodily features, as our functions become more acute and we move from a state of relative placidity to one of ecstatic surrender.

Of amorous submission.

Of impassioned pleasure.

Of wild abandon.

This change is the way of erotic love.

The look in one's eyes.

The subtle movement of bodies.

The moistening of lips.

The shift in stance.

The glistening of perspiration.

No.

The glistening of sweat.

Steamy.

Hot.

As you explore.

Discover.

Savour.

> 'WHAT I DO,
> AND WHAT I DREAM INCLUDES THEE,
> AS THE WINE MUST TASTE,
> OF ITS OWN GRAPE.'
>   Elizabeth Barrett Browning

All that is of the other.

And yourself.

Ourselves.

As individuals, unique.

In our duality, even more so.

For when we combine our life force with our beloved, we become a single entity of energy.

Call it karma.

Call it psychic.

Call it teamwork.

Call it awesome.

In its power to heal.

To inspire.

And to change.

The whole is greater than the sum of its parts. Yet the sum of the parts is whole.

Timeless proverbs imparting common knowledge? Yes, but such truths exemplify the way we are.

When next you become deeply intimate with your lover, consider where you are and how you feel with each other.

Observe the feelings and the combination of your energies.

As an example of this energetic connection, try these exercises with your beloved.

Sit cross-legged facing each other so that your knees are touching.

Hold each other's hands. Right hand facing down. Left hand facing up.

Gaze into each other's eyes.

Now go through the breathing routine of imagining the flow of air coming up through the centre of your body and flowing out the same way.

> 'HARMONY MAKES SMALL THINGS GROW;
> LACK OF IT MAKES GREAT THINGS DECAY.'
> Sallust

By getting into the pattern of both breathing simultaneously you will build up a surprising level of energy between you. When this happens, simply surrender to any feelings that come up.

Once you are comfortable breathing together, you can increase the level of intimacy with the man sitting cross-legged and the woman sitting on his lap. In this position, your bodies should be touching with your arms around each other.

By breathing together, allow your thoughts to come into the moment. To where you are and what you are doing. Get lost in the feelings, as the energy connection between you and your beloved starts to happen.

Ultimately, with a little practice, you can alternate your breathing so that one inhales as the other exhales.

There is no time limit on doing these exercises. They can be done for as little as five minutes or, if you sink into a state of meditation, as much as several hours. They can also be done with or without penetration.

For the man, if at any time you feel aroused to the point of ejaculation, simply ask your partner to stop and continue breathing deeply; otherwise remain still until the feeling subsides.

In fact, in any part of your sexual activities, it is OK to ask the other to stop. When you do, just relax into the feeling and stay in tune with each other.

Another variation on the previous exercise is circular breathing.

Upon inhalation, the man imagines his breath coming in through his heart and circling around to go out through his penis.

The woman imagines the reverse: the breath coming in through her vagina and out via her heart.

To get the full benefit of this, you will need to get your alternate breathing right.

All it takes is a little concentration and a little practice.

The more you get into the rhythm, the more you will notice the power growing between you.

Your oneness.

Surrounding you.

Encompassing you.

Drawing you into union.

It may come in waves or it may surge up and down your

spine, or it may encompass the two of you in a circle of light.

The subtle shift in your erotic energy will take you to a greater level of intimacy.

For you are together even when you are not. Allowing the other the space to be apart. To be alone.

And in aloneness the connection is always there.

But togetherness is not something to think about. When it happens, allow it to flow.

Too much thought gets in the way.

For this is the beginning of ecstasy. And ecstasy doesn't come from the head.

It comes from the heart.

EXPLORATION

To search out new frontiers.

To go where no person has gone before.

This, then, is the essence of exploration.

To encounter those parts of your partner's body that you haven't seen or touched before. Or have seen or touched only with trepidation.

Through our past conditioning, whether parental, religious or social, we all grow up with certain inhibitions.

In order for us to realise our full and total sensuality, it is these blockages that have to be broken down.

Obviously, the more private the part, the greater the boundary.

From your own perspective, there may be parts of your body that for one reason or another have never been touched by another person. Conversely, there may be areas of your beloved's body that you have never touched.

> 'I AM AN EXPLORER THEN, AND I AM ALSO A STALKER OR THE INSTRUMENT OF THE HUNT ITSELF.'
>
> Annie Dillard

After all, exploration is a two-way street.

You have to feel comfortable being the explorer as well as being the explored.

However, the path to you becoming a more sensual and erotic being does have that element of risk. It is by taking risks that you will emerge much more in tune with yourself and much more open to others.

Before entering any pleasuring or massage session with your partner, consider those parts of your body that you feel sensitive about. Those areas you have put restrictions on.

Lie still and close your eyes, focusing on those parts.

Connect with what you are feeling in relation to that aspect of your body that you have difficulty opening up to.

Ask yourself why it is that this part of your body is vulnerable. Why is it afraid to be touched or kissed?

It may be that you feel ashamed.

Or embarrassed.

Or shy.

Or confused.

Or guilty.

Or vulnerable.

If it is any one or more of these feelings, just stay with the emotion. And keep breathing into that area of the body you don't feel comfortable with.

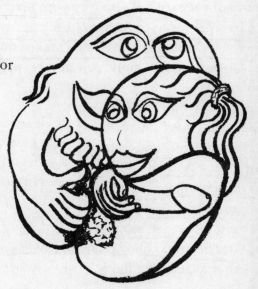

When you are ready to explore or be explored, open up one of your boundaries to your beloved. Take that chance. It is all part of the adventure.

For as that secret part of your body becomes exposed, then touched, then caressed, then nurtured, you will feel a new aliveness creep into your being.

This aliveness is the awakening of your sensuality.

As you breathe into each other's touch.

Each other's discovery.

This is the ultimate outcome of exploration.

For the more you look, the more you will find.

Pearls.

Gems.

A garden of untold erotic treasures.

A world of pleasurable delicacies.

A universe of ecstatic wonders.

May your search reap bountiful rewards.

> 'A DAY IN SUCH SERENE ENJOYMENT SPENT,
> IS WORTH AN AGE OF SPLENDID DISCONTENT.'
> James Montgomery

THE IMPORTANCE
OF SKIN

A learned scholar once alluded to skin as being vitally important because of the simple fact that it kept your insides in.

This, of course, is true.

Your skin, after all, is the largest organ in the body.

It breathes.

It feels.

It protects.

It eliminates.

It smells.

It perspires.

It absorbs.

It glows.

The significance of skin cannot be underestimated. Especially when it comes to intimacy.

Our skin is a unique and wonderful thing.

Stroke it and it feels warm and languid.

Smack it and it feels pain.

Run a feather lightly down it and it shivers.

Wrap your arms around it and it feels secure.

Massage it and it feels tender.

As we did when we were babies in allowing ourselves to experience the pleasure and sensations of our bodies.

We can survive without sight and sound. But take away touch also and the world will become barren.

Studies have shown that the emotional growth factor of a baby is directly linked to the way they are touched.

The next time you see a baby, observe how, in their innocence, they enjoy the wonder of touching and playing with themselves. Sadly, from an early age we are told that playing with ourselves is taboo. Yet being comfortable and free within our body is vitally important in the way we develop our sensuality.

> 'I'VE GOT YOU, UNDER MY SKIN.'
> Cole Porter

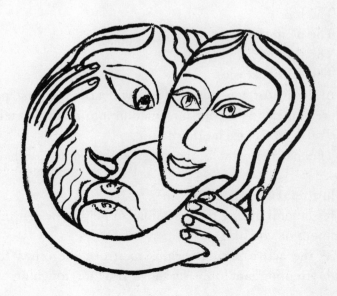

Note also the way a baby loves to be touched and stroked. The squeals of delight. The giggling. The languid drifting into sleep.

In truth, these desires and sensations remain with us always.

Skin is a remarkable aphrodisiac. Even before you touch it, the simple perusing of skin can be a highly erotic and sensual experience.

While I have previously talked about looking lovingly at your beloved's body, this exercise is more specific.

Sit naked with your partner, looking into each other's eyes.

Slowly run your gaze over their skin.

Behold the softness.

The folds.

The freckles.

The hair.

The blemishes.

The colour.

The idiosyncrasies.

After five or ten minutes you will arrive at that point where you can turn your imagination into reality by taking it in turns to feel each other's skin.

The partner who is the receiver lies down with eyes closed.

Just relax and keep breathing.

It's helpful during these sessions to play some soft music that both of you like.

As the active partner begins to stroke the other, focus your attention not only on how you are touching your beloved, but also on becoming the touch. Allow yourself to experience yourself in the giving, just as your beloved is experiencing themself in the receiving.

Tune in to the pristine beauty of your beloved's skin and imagine all the things you can do to it.

Then do them.

Caress the skin.

Lick it.

Kiss it.

Fondle it.

Smell it.

Nuzzle it.

Breathe on it.

Squeeze it.

Bite it.

Embrace it.

And become it.

Isn't skin amazing?

After about 30 minutes change places.

When you have both finished, have a hot bath together. Rub soap over each other. Splash water. Kiss and caress your wet skin. Then each dry the other. Feeling the sensation of the towel over your body.

> 'COME LIVE WITH ME, AND BE MY LOVE,
> AND WE WILL SOME NEW PLEASURES PROVE,
> OF GOLDEN SANDS, AND CRYSTAL BROOKS,
> WITH SILKEN LINES, AND SILVER HOOKS.'
>
> John Donne

Before you get into bed, stand looking into each other's eyes.

Give each other a long, sensuous hug.

Skin to skin.

Now, climb into bed.

Replete in the discovery that love is more than skin deep.

And you thought that all skin did was keep your insides in!

> 'WHENEVER YOU ARE
> SINCERELY PLEASURED, YOU ARE
> NOURISHED.'
>> Ralph Waldo Emerson

THE MAGIC
OF MASSAGE

WHEN it comes to exploring the body of your beloved, feeling the beauty and texture of their skin, then it is natural for you to turn your mind to the ancient art of massage.

Massage is one of the most precious gifts a person can bestow upon another.

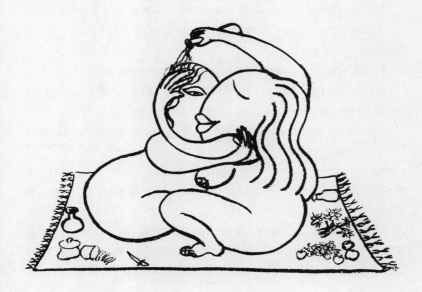

It is touch at its most sensory and sensual.

Playful and passionate.

Earthy and erotic.

Massage in the context of intimacy can be about as intimate as you can get.

It all depends on how you give it.

And receive it.

To run your hands over the body of your lover can be a very special part of your relationship.

To press the flesh.

To stroke it.

To squeeze it.

To tantalise it.

To tease it.

To nurture it.

The one thing to remember always is that to massage your beloved is an extension of your love.

For in many ways, massage goes beyond sex, because for it to really work, you virtually have to surrender your entire body to your partner.

However, for many people this may pose some difficulty.

As discussed earlier, initially there may be a number of areas of your body that are sensitive to the touch of another. If this is the case, then, prior to a massage session, discuss openly with your partner what you want and don't want. By communicating your boundaries in this way you will be strengthening the bond of trust and honesty between yourselves.

Conversely, crossing those boundaries, by allowing your body to be lightly and sensitively touched in those areas that are sensitive, can be extremely healing. You will be surprised at how the more risk you take, the more your relationship will be enhanced.

Before your massage, set up your special space. Ensure that it is really comfortable, with candles and incense and soft, relaxing music.

Make sure you have a really good massage oil. Baby oil will not do. The oil you use should be a quality massage oil, such as apricot kernel oil or almond oil that are available at either new age shops, some quality whole food stores or specialist outlets. These oils are edible, which gives you the freedom to kiss or lick your partner during the massage, should you so desire.

You can buy preformulated massage oil or a plain base oil and scent it yourself with essential oils such as patchouli, ylang-ylang, sandalwood or orange. Or whatever scent pleases you.

Avoid using oils packaged in plastic bottles as they tend to absorb the filler from the plastic, which can be harmful to some sensitive skins.

> 'THE WHOLE PLEASURE OF LOVE LIES IN THE VARIETY.'
> Molière

It is best to keep the oil warm whether by keeping the bottle or container in a bowl of hot water or by placing it on or near a heater.

Once you have the oil under control, nominate who is going to be the receiver and who is going to be the giver.

The receiver's job is to do nothing but give their body over to the unknown.

The way to begin is for the giver to lead their partner to the special place. Help them to lie face down, making sure they are as comfortable as possible with pillows under their head and legs.

After you, as the receiver, have set your boundaries, allow yourself to be taken without resistance.

When you are lying down, let yourself go. As you do, breathe in the aromas, the ambience and the surroundings.

Focus on where your partner's hands are and what they are doing.

Just be with it.

Remember that one word: *surrender*.

During the massage, it's OK for you as the receiver to make sounds of pleasure if something feels good. At the same time, do not be afraid to ask your partner to continue or discontinue doing something that you may or may not be enjoying. You can do this by a gentle hand movement.

The giver needs to be aware that there is no need to rush – that they can take all the time in the world.

You have nothing to do and nowhere to go.

There is no hard and fast rule about what part of the body you should start to massage first. However, because the front of the body has a number of sensitive areas, starting with the back will allow your partner to relax into the massage earlier.

Here is a suggested massage routine that you can vary, improve or change in whichever way best fits how you and your partner feel.

As giver, when you touch your beloved, do not focus on the touch but become the touch.

Be at one with the touch.

For, in so doing, your love, your energy and your whole being will emanate from your hands.

Commence by softly placing the palms of your hands on the soles of your partner's feet. Leave them there for a few minutes, closing your eyes, directing your energy and feelings into your hands.

Then put one hand on the small of the back and the other between the shoulder blades. Close your eyes and as you exhale, imagine your love extending out through your hands.

After a few minutes, very slowly lift the hands off the back.

Once you have released your hands, pour some oil into them and rub them together. Now run your hands down your partner's back and buttocks in order to spread the oil, slowly working them over their back, bit by bit.

> 'GOOD LOVERS HAVE KNOWN FOR CENTURIES THAT THE HAND IS PROBABLY THE PRIMARY SEX ORGAN.'
> Eleanor Hamilton

In massage, versatility is the key.

Squeeze your partner's flesh between your fingers.

Rub it gently.

Be firm.

Be gentle.

Then let your fingers flutter very lightly from their neck down to their buttocks.

Be creative with the direction and motion of your hands.

> 'MY HANDS ARE MY PENIS.'
> Mickey Rourke

For most people, having their buttocks massaged is an extremely pleasurable experience. Just continue stroking in

...e same way as you have done with the back. It is with the buttocks or the top of the legs that you may well incur the most likely boundary: How far do you go? The answer to this is: As far as you're allowed.

Always remember, the more you explore, the greater the thrill.

So take a risk.

Let your fingers go where they will and do what feels right and you and your beloved will both have a wonderful experience.

> 'IF YOU DON'T RISK ANYTHING, YOU RISK EVEN MORE.'
>
> Erica Jong

The buttocks can be returned to, after you have done the legs, which follow the same basic pattern as the back.

Don't forget the toes.

One at a time.

And the soles of the feet.

Run your hands around each leg and up and down them. Especially the inner thigh, which for many people is quite sensitive.

After you have completed the legs you can return to the buttocks by including them as part of the leg routine. Then run your hands all over your beloved's body.

If you feel the urge, allow them to feel the pleasure of your body by lying on them and moving your body over them. This closeness can be extremely delicious.

During the massage you will probably feel a strong desire to kiss and caress your beloved's body. Do this with softness and genuine feeling.

Become the kiss.

Become the caress.

If at this time, either of you become aroused, allow the sensation to be.

Just focus on what you're feeling and how you're feeling it. And keep breathing deeply.

Upon completing massaging the back, lightly kiss your beloved's cheek and ear lobe and sensuously whisper into their ear that it is <u>time for them to turn over.</u>

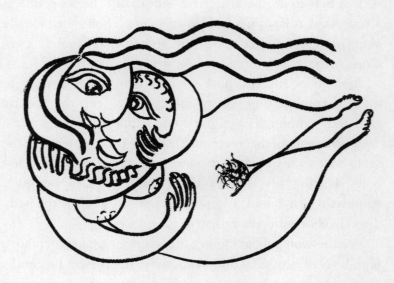

This is easier than it sounds, because, depending on the way you have massaged the back, turning over will take quite an effort.

Sit back and allow your beloved the time and space to make the move. There is no need for them to rush.

Eventually they will slowly muster the energy to roll over and when they do, make sure you are there to help them.

When they are lying on their back, place one hand on their heart and the other on their stomach, just above the navel. Allow them to settle down, while you close your eyes and direct your energy and love into their body.

Encourage your beloved to breathe deeply, focusing on letting go with each exhalation.

After a few minutes slowly release your hands.

It is now time to return to the massage.

It is best to do the arms first. Simply lift them up, one at a time, and rub oil up and down them. Then move slowly along each section: the upper arm, forearm, wrists and hands. Don't forget the fingers.

Remember, the purpose of this massage is simply to nurture your partner, not to achieve any deep therapeutic catharsis – although anything could happen.

If the man is the receiver, then his front is treated the same way as his back. Run your hands over the chest and belly. Having his nipples lightly touched can be quite stimulating for a man, as can having the area below the belly directly above the genitals stroked.

For the woman, having her breasts massaged can create a high level of arousal. Unless otherwise instructed, be gentle. Slowly run your hands over the breasts, lightly squeezing them and teasing the nipples. The receiver should make sure to let their partner know what feels good.

Don't forget that the belly also contains much of a woman's power and sensitivity.

Massaging the legs from the front is the same basic procedure as doing them from the back. Don't forget the feet, toes and inner thigh.

Which brings us to the genitals.

Some people, when it comes to being massaged, prefer that their genitals are not touched. In the case of sensual massage, by the time you get to this area it is highly likely there will be quite a deal of arousal.

The way you touch your lover's genitals is one of individual preference.

Be guided by each other.

Tell the other what you like and what feels good, as well as what doesn't.

Many men fear having an erection and try to suppress it. Don't.

If your penis decides to rise to the occasion, then allow it to do so. It would be unusual for a woman not to like to see an erect penis.

At this point it can be easy to lose control over the massage. If either or both of you feel a strong desire to let yourselves go, hold on.

And keep breathing.

Allow the feelings to circulate within your bodies.

Remain in the space you have created and stay with what you are doing.

There are no goals to be reached. You are simply being at one with your beloved. Whatever occurs will happen in its own way.

'ALL WHICH SPIRITUALLY LAYS CLAIM ON A MAN GOES TO THE SENSES; THEREFORE, IS IT THAT THROUGH THEM HE FEELS HIMSELF MOVED TO ALL THINGS?'

Bettina von Arnim

The final area to massage is the face and head. Both are acutely sensitive to touch, and the more emotive you are, the deeper the sensation will be. Massaging this area last is a way of centring the recipient.

The face should be done with care as, for many people, the face is the area of most sensitivity. You can use your hands, fingers, tongue or lips to lightly roam all over it. The forehead, nose, eyes, ears, neck, lips. Languidly press and caress each part.

Run your fingers through your partner's hair and around the base of their neck.

At the end of the session, lie down next to your beloved and simply be with them. Gently stroke their hair or chest or stomach.

When the time is right, sit up and face each other.

The receiving partner thanks the giver for nurturing and honouring their body. While the giver thanks the receiver for allowing them to enter their space and for accepting their love.

Bow to each other and give each other a deep hug.

You may now like to share a hot, aromatic bath.

It is a good idea, but not mandatory, for only one massage to occur at a time. Allow a day to reverse the roles.

As you will discover, massage is a very important and sensitive way to unify a relationship.

Massage also offers all the high erotica of sex beyond intercourse. As such, it can be a sensual encounter that is measured in hours rather than minutes.

Why not break out the oil today?

SHARING WATER

ONE of the well-known dictums espoused by the conservation movement when urging the populace to conserve water is that we should shower with a friend.

This is an appealing concept, as more often than not the friend in question is also our lover.

The sharing of water is one of life's more intimate experiences.

> 'NOBLE DEEDS AND HOT BATHS ARE THE BEST CURE FOR DEPRESSION.'
> Dodie Smith

Both bathing and showering together have their own unique aspects.

If you are planning to make love, then it is best to have a bath before such a liaison, as it not only cleanses the body but can arouse and stimulate.

If you are giving or receiving a massage, then having a bath after the session is an extremely grounding experience, because of its ability to relax and nurture.

Your first task prior to your bath is to turn the bathroom into a special place by positioning candles strategically around the room. Then fill the bath with warm water, sprinkling a few drops of aromatic oil in it. As with the blending of your massage oils, a combination of sandalwood, patchouli, orange or ylang-ylang are the most suitable. However, there may well be some other fragrances that you like.

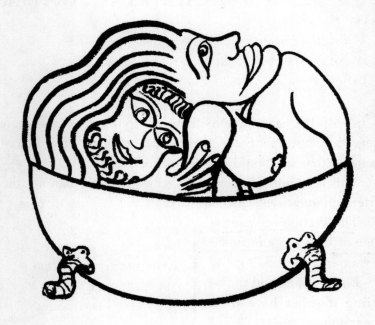

Scatter a few flower petals over the water.

If you have access to a sound system, soft, sensual music will also enhance the experience.

On entering the bathroom each disrobes the other so that you are looking at each other's naked bodies by the light of the candles.

After a few minutes, give each other a long, lingering hug before getting into the bath.

Because most baths are relatively small, the first time you share the experience it may take you some time to work out the best positions. These can vary from lying facing each other to one of you lying along the other with your back against the other's chest to, if you're really adventurous, lying one on top of the other.

The idea is that once you are settled, you should remain relatively still.

Allow the water to circulate around your bodies.

Inhale the aroma of the bath oils.

After a while, you may wish to rub soap over your beloved.

Or sensuously nibble their toes.

Or playfully splash water at each other.

Or just hold each other, feeling the moisture, the wetness of the other's body.

Eventually, the time will come when you will need to move on. (Usually when the water gets cold or your fingers become wrinkled!)

> 'I FEEL ABOUT A HOT BATH THE WAY RELIGIOUS PEOPLE FEEL ABOUT HOLY WATER.'
> Sylvia Plath

Slowly, both of you get out of the bath and wrap yourselves in fluffy towels.

You can give each other another hug while drying off.

It is best to keep your post-bath activity on a much more spiritual level.

You may choose to be in your special place or fall into bed and just be with each other.

Inhaling the sweet clean smell of the other and exploring the softness of their skin.

Like newborn babies.

Curled up in each other's arms.

To love.
To sleep.
To dream.

Showering together works best in the morning, especially after a night of intimate abandon.

There is something really erotic about holding your lover with water cascading all over you.

A shower adds the finishing touch.

Rubbing soap over each other.

Letting your fingers find their way to all those places where fingers like to find themselves.

To kiss passionately with warm water streaming down your faces and over your lips and into your mouths.

To press each other against the wall of the shower.

Pressing. Pressing.

Feeling the wet and sensuous lines of each other's body.

This first rite of the day now takes on a new perspective.

As you dry off and move into the morning.

Apart or together.

Remaining connected.

As lovers always do.

> 'FISH FUCK IN IT.'
> W. C. Fields

IGNITING
THE FLAME

Arousal.

The feeling that can arise at any time.

In any place.

With anybody.

Or somebody.

When you least expect it.

As you gaze into another's eyes.

Or hug.

Or stroke their body.

An inner stirring begins to awaken.

Of want.

Of longing.

Of anticipation.

This is the spark of desire.

That burst of internal combustion.

That harnessing of your sexual energy.

Your aliveness.

As the juices start to flow.

As this feeling starts to take hold, allow your breath to connect with it.

And when you do, let yourself surrender to the feelings.

For this is the precursor.

To the pleasure that is happening and to the delights on the horizon.

This is ignition.

Lift-off.

And it will be your energy and that of your partner that will take you into orbit.

An energy, a power, a flame that is difficult to extinguish.

If not impossible.

> 'PLEASURE IS VERY SELDOM
> FOUND WHERE IT IS SOUGHT;
> OUR BRIGHTEST BLAZES OF
> GLADNESS ARE COMMONLY
> KINDLED BY UNEXPECTED
> SPARKS.'
>
> Samuel Johnson

THE ALCHEMY
OF HONESTY

THROUGHOUT our lives, whether it is with ourselves or with others, we are continually playing games with our emotional honesty.

In many ways, we tend to mask our true feelings and hide our secrets.

What, in fact, we are doing is keeping all of our pain, anger and frustration locked away deep inside us, which deadens the experience of our sensuality.

Despite this, we still manage to put on a brave face.

When asked how we are feeling, we invariably reply, 'Good'.

Good?

How good?

By what degree?

Or is it, perhaps, not really that good?

In truth, we would probably feel good if this, that or the other occurred.

We may come into some money.

We may get a new job.

We may start a new relationship.

But, whether or not any of these do occur, we are relying on superficial aspects to improve our lives, while our emotional outlook remains unchanged.

> 'IF WE BE HONEST WITH OURSELVES,
> WE SHALL BE HONEST WITH OTHERS.'
> George MacDonald

So we continue to live in the anticipation that we will be feeling good, sometime in the foreseeable future, providing something happens to us that will be the catalyst to some uplifting of our disposition.

From a personal perspective, you really need to stop your forward momentum, in order to give yourself enough time to reflect on what it is that's really happening to you.

To acknowledge the truth about yourself, to yourself.

And to your beloved.

Accepting who you are and the fact that you really only exist in this moment.

We too often dwell on the past and anticipate the future. Because you don't live in either aspect, neither has any relevance.

> 'I LOVE YOU MORE THAN
> YESTERDAY, BUT NOT AS
> MUCH AS TOMORROW.'
> Edmond Rostand

If, when confronted by fear or anxiety, you bring your mind back to exactly where you are and what you are doing at this instant, this moment, you will find that the importance of the situation is lessened.

It is this perspective that allows you to expand the parameters of your honesty.

By finally arriving in the moment, you will discover that it is the acceptance of honesty that is one of the prime ingredients within a truly loving relationship.

Honesty that is given without recrimination.

Honesty that is shared with love.

Honesty that is about revealing, to your partner, those secrets or disappointments or irritations or desires that you have in your life.

Openly and without holding back.

Especially those deep, dark secrets that only you and your teddy bear know.

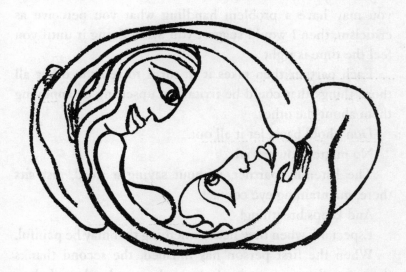

And sharing a deep, dark secret with someone may well unlock one of your greatest fears. That once you've told them, they will probably say something like 'So?' It is at this point that you will come to the realisation that it wasn't much of a secret after all, simply because the only person judging it was you.

Revealing yourself to your beloved in this way is an intrinsic part of a loving and intimate relationship.

Here is an exercise that you can do every now and then. Once a month would be ideal, although you may feel the need to do it on a more regular basis. Before you start, you should be aware that this exercise has a number of uses.

Ideally, it is an opening up to each other and in this context is not designed to start an argument. Conversely, if either one of you feels you have a number of issues to discuss, then this process can circumvent an argument.

Just stay tuned to each other and if you feel that inwardly you may have a problem handling what you perceive as criticism, then I would suggest you avoid doing it until you feel the time is right.

Each partner then takes it in turns to tell the other all those things that could be irritating, upsetting or annoying them about the other.

Don't hold back, let it all out.

No matter how trivial.

The listening partner, without saying a word, just sits there, maintaining eye contact.

And keeps breathing!

Especially when they hear something that may be painful.

When the first person has finished, the second thanks them for sharing a part of themselves and acknowledges what they had to say. They should not comment or argue about any point that may have caused them to feel angry or anxious.

Then the roles are reversed.

Be aware that as the listener you do not take on what the other person is

'HE THAT LOSETH HIS HONESTY, HAS NOTHING LEFT TO LOSE.'

John Lyly

saying as a form of criticism. While it may appear that you are being unjustly accused or dumped upon, this, in fact, is not the case.

Criticism is often the domain of the criticiser.

Just remember to keep breathing and to let the words settle and then wash away. It is the letting go that is important.

When you have completed this process, for sixty seconds each partner tells the other something about themselves that they hadn't revealed to the other. This could be a desire, some incident out of their past, an embarrassing moment, how much money they have in the bank, a secret disease. Anything. Just keep talking for sixty seconds. On completion, the listening partner thanks the other for sharing their secret.

Now each of you reveal to your beloved all those positive aspects you feel about them. It could be the way they talk, their mannerisms, something they may have done that appealed to you. Don't be embarrassed, just let your feelings flow. Again, you give each other acknowledgement and thank them for sharing a part of themselves.

Finally, after each has had a turn, the two of you sit quietly and discuss any of the revelations that were brought up. But don't prolong it. If any of what is said is justified, simply acknowledge it and move on.

Then close your eyes, each bowing down in honour of yourself and your beloved.

Now open your eyes and look at each other.

See the beauty, the feelings, the love and the honesty.

And in the seeing, feel the beauty, the love and the honesty.

Now both give each other a long, lingering hug and climb into bed.

What you will have discovered, is a new-found connection to your loved one.

You have been drawn closer together by a mutual sharing and revealing of secrets that are unique to you. You now know something new about your beloved and have given something of yourself that you haven't previously shared.

Not just from a sexual perspective, but from every aspect of your lives.

For while honesty is a vital component of any relationship, it need not be confined to just one person. Every day we experience a closeness with those around us with whom we interact on a regular basis. Because of this, the same precepts of honesty hold true, whether it is with yourself or with another.

It is this honesty that will enrich your relationships beyond belief.

> 'I WILL HAVE NO LOCKED
> CUPBOARDS IN MY LIFE.'
> Gertrude Bell

WHAT'S GOING ON
INSIDE YOUR HEAD?

PLENTY.

And none of it has to do with what it is you are doing.
Or feeling.

Especially when it comes to sex.

This is because we are
conditioned to live inside
our heads, to look at things
from an analytical per-
spective, and it is this that
invariably constricts our emotional and sensual growth.

> 'THE HEART IS WISER THAN
> THE INTELLECT.'
> J. G. Holland

This is not to suggest that we shouldn't be analytical. It's
just that, at times, our heads conjure up thoughts, criticisms,
excuses, reactions, evaluations, questions, opinions, assump-
tions, judgements and a whole lot of other clutter that stands
in the way of our finding true emotional equilibrium.

It is this continuous chatter that we need to control, in
order to get our consciousness out of our heads and into our
bodies.

And our hearts.

If you don't think it's true about living inside your head, here's an exercise you can try with your partner. Like all the processes in this book it requires absolute honesty.

Lie down next to each other, either in your special place or on your bed.

Clothing is optional.

This exercise is taken in turns, with one of you doing the talking and the other the listening.

Whoever is first, lie on your back while your partner lies on their side close to you, placing their hand at the centre of your chest, the heart centre in the body that controls your feelings of compassion and consciousness..

Close your eyes and take a number of deep breaths. With each exhalation, allow your body to sink deeper into the mattress.

Start to visualise a typical sexual experience either with or without your beloved.

This scenario should be all the aspects leading up to sexual activity, as well as during and after. Allow the flow of those thoughts that normally come into your head while making love.

> 'WHERE THE HEAD IS PAST HOPE, THE HEART IS PAST SHAME.'
>
> John Lyly

As each image or desire comes to mind, say it, out loud. Everything.

The apprehensions, the doubts, the anticipation, the hopes, the feelings, the desires.

The grocery list, the football scores, the bills, your mother, your father, your workload and so on.

Various positions you'd like to be doing it in.

Places you want your partner to touch, lick, fondle, scratch, pull, poke, suck and kiss.

Everything.

Don't hold back.

Let it all hang out.

And don't stop until you're finished.

The more you let go of the truth, the better you are going to feel.

If you are doing the listening you should just be with your beloved, being aware of what they are going through and what they are feeling.

Also be aware of the cathartic nature of this experience.

At the end of the process, just lie together, holding each other.

When the time feels right, thank your beloved for allowing you to share your thoughts. The other simply acknowledges their partner's honesty.

You will then change places and repeat the exercise.

What this process serves to demonstrate is that once you get out of your heads and into your hearts, then you will truly start to get in touch with your emotions and your sexuality.

You will discover a renewed innocence and playfulness emerging in your lovemaking. By becoming more present, and in the moment, you will not be cutting off parts of yourself from your lover.

The more you express what you want, the more you will be fulfilled.

Your heart never lies.

Only your head is capable of that.

> 'I LOVE THEE FOR A HEART
> THAT'S KIND, NOT FOR THE
> KNOWLEDGE IN THY MIND.'
> W. H. Davies

THE DELUSION
OF FANTASY

IN erotic love there is no such thing as fantasy. Not in the true meaning of the word.

The term fantasy literally means dreams that are unobtainable.

Visions that are relatively abstract.

Illusions that are totally improbable.

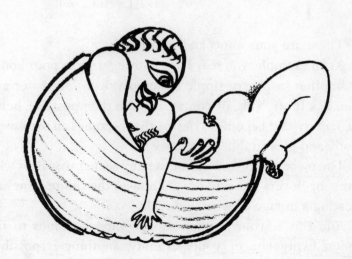

A fantasy may constitute the scenario of making love to a *Penthouse* centrefold, a sports hero or a movie star. It could be to make love in a public place or to create a situation that would be impossible to manifest. The maxim is that in the remote possibility of bringing any of these episodes to life, they will not, in any way, be as imagined.

Fantasies can also include those acts of offbeat or unusual sexual endeavours you would like to participate in with your partner or partners. However, because these concepts have a greater chance of coming to fruition, they do not necessarily fall into the realm of fantasy.

> 'CHILD OF THE PURE UNCLOUDED BROW
> AND DREAMING EYES OF WONDER,
> THOUGH TIME BE FLEET AND I AND THOU
> ARE HALF A LIFE ASUNDER,
> THY LOVING SMILE WILL SURELY HAIL
> THE LOVE-GIFT OF A FAIRY-TALE.'
>
> Lewis Carroll

These are your wants and your needs.

As an example, you may have a strong urge to pour honey or smother raspberry ripple ice-cream over your lover and then lick it off. This, of course, is more than possible, being the fantasy that becomes a desire, that becomes an extremely erotic and pleasurable experience.

The more you dream of hot, steamy sexual scenarios with lover or lovers known or unknown, the more you are creating a mirage of what you really want.

And this is your truth, because when it comes to the honest expression of your sexuality, anything is possible, provided both you and your partner are in agreement.

If agreement is not forthcoming, then the ensuing disagreement will be manifested as denial. This means that what you want you can't have, and if the only way to get it is in your dreams, so be it. When you are in this state of denial or you have an inability to give of yourself, the more frequent and greater your fantasies become because fantasy is a product of denial.

The problem with continued fantasies is that they cover up underlying problems within your relationship and, as such, are another way of taking your head to bed.

The more you are present when making love, the more total the experience, the more connected you will be to your beloved. There is no need for fantasy while you stay in the moment; the greatest fantasy of all is being intimate with each other.

Consequently, because of its ability to bring you into the moment and into your being, when you experience the totality of orgasm, fantasy no longer exists.

Only the reality.

> 'THE DESIRES OF THE HEART ARE
> AS CROOKED AS CORKSCREWS.'
>
> W. H. Auden

EXERCISE
TO ECSTASY

WHILE much of sex beyond intercourse lies in the aspect of sensuality and spirituality, it is still important to have one's body in tune.

This doesn't mean that you should be a triathlete, but the fitter you are, the greater your stamina will be.

Whatever your level of fitness, there is one muscle in the body that is vital to maintaining your sexual energy.

This muscle is known as the pubococcygeus, or PC muscle for short.

The PC muscle is situated between the genitals and the anus. It is the muscle you squeeze when you need to control the flow of urine.

When next you're urinating, stop the flow in midstream.

Voila! You've just found your PC muscle.

From a sexual perspective, it is the PC muscle that first comes into play when you have an orgasm. For this reason, being aware of and in control of the PC muscle can greatly improve and prolong orgasm.

For a man, with the help of practice and breathing, the PC muscle actually assists in curtailing ejaculation.

It is relatively easy to exercise and strengthen the PC muscle. You can do it just lying on a bed or on the floor. And you don't need a partner, although you can do it together.

Simply relax your whole body.

Bend your knees.

Now, squeeze the PC muscle in and out. As you would when you urinate.

Once you get the hang of that, you can lift your hips forward and back as in a pelvic thrust. Concentrate on the area of the PC muscle as you inhale on the forward motion, exhaling as you release.

And if you start to feel pleasurable, go with it.

Flexing your PC muscle is not meant to be hard work.

You can do this procedure for five to ten minutes a day or whenever the urge strikes you.

Another important exercise brings in the whole pelvic area.

It is called The Wave

To do The Wave, stand relaxed, with your legs at shoulder width apart.

To the count of four, move your pelvis forward, upward, and back as if it is turning on a wheel.

As you come over the top, inhale, and as you push through the bottom, exhale. Your arms also move in a circular motion by your side, in line with the pelvis.

Try to keep the rest of your body still.

As you get into the rhythm, you will start to gain fluidity.

The Wave can be practised alone with eyes closed or facing a partner while holding eye contact.

Finding a piece of music that has a continuous beat can greatly enhance this exercise. One album that is good to do The Wave to is *Shamanic Dream* (Nightingale NGH-CD-321).

Doing The Wave for fifteen to twenty minutes will intensify the feeling in your pelvic area. Allow this to happen, remembering to breathe deeply into it.

The Wave can also be done lying down or on your hands and knees.

Keeping the PC muscle and pelvis in shape, as well as your whole body, is important in maintaining better control over your sexuality.

Which is something worth raising a sweat over.

SELF-PLEASURE
THROUGH MEDITATION

ONCE you have become totally comfortable with your body on both a spiritual and physical level, you can then allow yourself to go through a self-pleasuring experience simply by meditating and breathing.

> 'WHY NOT SEIZE THE PLEASURE AT ONCE? HOW OFTEN IS HAPPINESS DESTROYED BY PREPARATION, FOOLISH PREPARATION!'
>
> Jane Austen

This, of course, goes beyond masturbation, because it allows you to connect and hold your orgasmic energy.

For a man this is especially important, because masturbation usually means self-stimulation until ejaculation. What this may do is elicit a let-down feeling and, in many instances, feelings of guilt.

Meditative self-pleasure allows you to bring yourself to ecstasy without the downside.

For a woman, as well as a man, meditating into an orgasmic release will result in a prolonged period of pleasure.

Lie on your bed with your eyes closed.

With each exhalation, feel your body sink deeper into the mattress.

Clear your mind of all outside thoughts.

Keep breathing deep into your belly.

Let your awareness slowly work its way around your body. Toes, legs, chest, arms, hands, neck, head and face.

Now, focus your mind on the area around your genitals.

Shift your breathing so that you imagine your breath being drawn up through your genitals and exhaled the same way. Allow the PC muscle to draw in and out with the breath.

After a while, you may start to detect a slight pulse through the pelvic area. Keep your mind focused on this.

Once you are in tune with the pulsation, start to increase the rapidity of your breathing. Keep squeezing the PC muscle. You may start to feel like moving your pelvis and hips up and down.

Imagine a hollow tube running up the centre of your body. As you inhale, feel the breath flowing in through your genitals, streaming up through the tube. Initially you may only be able to feel it as high as your abdomen or chest. However, once you've had some practice, you will be able to draw the energy to your neck and out through the top of your head.

On the exhalation, release the PC muscle and allow the breath to flow back through the genital area.

You may start to experience a warm feeling in your genitals.

You may get the feeling that you are standing under a waterfall.

Your body may actually start vibrating.

You may even feel like quickening your breath. This, too, is encouraged.

Eventually, after some practice, you will be able to elevate the level of excitement until your breathing becomes almost like panting.

When this happens, the operative word again is *surrender.*

Upon reaching this point, just let go.

Whatever you are feeling, surrender to it.

Once you do, you will soon find your whole body moving uncontrollably.

Just allow whatever happens to happen. The entire feeling of pleasure surrounding you.

This sequence can last for minutes or even hours. As long as you want.

Men especially will find they will be able to enjoy this sensation without the need for ejaculation.

There will come a point when it will subside to a natural conclusion. When this occurs allow the breathing to slow down.

When your breathing returns to normal, just lie there feeling the sensations that are inside and outside your body.

Feel the aliveness and the power you have just generated.

'HOW DOES IT FEEL
TO BE ON YOUR OWN,
WITH NO DIRECTION HOME,
LIKE A COMPLETE UNKNOWN,
LIKE A ROLLING STONE?'

Bob Dylan

Feel the pleasure you have just given yourself.

Feel the love you have given yourself.

Feel the love of yourself.

THE LANGUAGE
OF LOVE

ONE of the most sensitive and vulnerable parts of our body is our ears.

Our sense of hearing captures much of the world's erotic and sensory delights.

As well as the distractions.

It is through the ears, as giver and receiver, that a unique ethereal bond is created.

> 'THE EAR IS THE ROAD TO
> THE HEART.'
>
> Voltaire

Your ears pick up more than you realise.

The next time you are walking through a park, stop and close your eyes and focus on all the noises. You will start to become aware of a multiplicity of different sounds that you have never noticed before.

The same is true when you are exploring your sensuality.

For many people, having their ears sucked and licked and breathed into is an exquisitely exciting experience.

For others, the language of love, spoken soft and low, imparts the same feelings.

It may also be the sound of a certain type of music that gets the internal juices flowing.

Or it may be the silence.

The silence that allows you to go within yourself and to be in your own time and space.

When you are with your beloved you need to open up your hearing to what is going on around you.

> 'HE WHO KNOWS, DOES NOT SPEAK, HE WHO SPEAKS, DOES NOT KNOW.'
> Lao-Tzu

The more you listen, the more intense the excitement.

The way your partner breathes.

The moans of ecstasy.

The screams of desire.

On the other hand, as your pleasure increases, you may wish to internalise and concentrate on being aware of your own inner feelings.

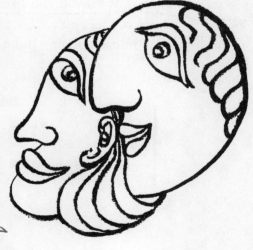

To give you an example, a simple game you can play is to each take it in turns to arouse each other's sense of hearing, with one being the giver and the other the receiver.

The receiver simply lies down, either blindfolded or with eyes closed. The giver arranges a series of aural delights using instruments or recorded sounds such as bells, rattles, drums, running water, music. One at a time, just run the sound around the other's head and down their body. Or just play it in one spot and let it envelop them. The giver can also, without saying a word, softly stroke the receiver's ears, breathe into them or lick them.

Towards the end, just stop and allow the silence to take over, for in silence there is connection. And after the hearing has been sensualised, the silence takes on a renewed significance.

The process need not take any more than ten to fifteen minutes. After you have both had a turn, sit facing each other and share your feelings about what you felt. Did the process stir your emotions? What did you like or dislike about the sounds? What are you feeling?

What you say to each other will be the best thing you'll hear all day.

> 'TO SPEAK OF LOVE
> IS TO MAKE LOVE.'
>   Honoré de Balzac

The sweet smell
of sensuality

IF ever there was a genuine aphrodisiac, it is body odour.
So it is paradoxical that the cosmetic industry, in their
infinite wisdom, has denounced body odour as unacceptable.

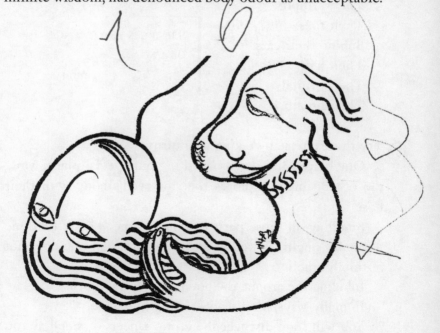

This is not to say that you need not wear fragrances; it is just that there is no real reason to cover up your true self either.

The way you smell is another facet of what and who you are.

To breathe in the aroma and nuances of your beloved can be an uplifting experience.

We all have our own particular smell, as we all have our own peculiar sense of smell. What doesn't smell pleasant to one person may actually attract another.

You could say that smell is in the nose of the sniffer.

Don't be afraid to explore and inhale all the warm and delicious places that are buried all over your lover's body.

All their nooks and crannies.

Their armpits.

Their toes.

Behind their ears.

Their hair.

Their genitals.

Their breath.

> 'DESIRE IS THE ESSENCE OF A MAN.'
>
> Spinoza

Try this exercise by taking it in turns.

One of you lies down naked in your special place, while the other simply explores their beloved's body with their nose.

Smelling all those parts of your partner's body that one normally smells, as well as all those parts that one does not normally smell.

Inhaling the aroma, the bouquet, the fragrance.

In many ways, it's just like tasting fine wine.

You will soon discover the erotic aspects of smell as you

take a little more risk by delving into those unseen areas, drawing in the unique odour that is inherent in your beloved.

At the same time, as you exhale, gently blow a stream of air onto your lover's skin as you share in what is by now becoming a mutually exciting and revealing experience.

After about fifteen to twenty minutes of breathing in the beauty of your lover, change places.

Aroma is a facet of intimacy that is often overlooked or not considered important. But, like all the senses, its role in creating arousal and deep passion cannot be underestimated.

Now you can breathe a little easier.

> 'THE SENSES ARE NOT DISCREET.'
>   Hannah Green

FUN WITH FOOD

IN a scene from the 1971 movie *Klute*, Jane Fonda is languidly following Donald Sutherland upstairs to their room in a small country hotel when she turns to the hotel reception clerk and asks him to 'send up a bottle of maple syrup'.

One wonders how many people at the time realised what use Fonda's character had in mind for the maple syrup. But it is a

> 'THE TORCH OF LOVE IS LIT IN THE KITCHEN.'
>
> French proverb

graphic example that when it comes to exploring creative sensuality, food can certainly enhance the experience.

As well as satisfying the hunger.

There are two basic principles to be followed when you introduce food as a part of your loveplay: to feed each other and to share bountifully.

You may initiate a session of fun with food, at a nominated meal time or as a part of making love.

Or both.

You will be surprised at the emotions and feelings that come up by being given food by your beloved.

Such is the playfulness that this process can generate, you may well find that you both become like children again.

> 'TELL ME WHAT YOU EAT, I'LL TELL YOU WHAT YOU ARE.'
> Brillat-Savarin

The seemingly simple routine of feeding another person and, in turn, being fed, can also generate a rare kind of nurturing.

If it is at the dinner table, you will both become giver and receiver of the repast. Each taking it in turns to put a piece of food into the other's mouth.

Sounds easy?

And you thought it was hard feeding a baby!

When it comes to dessert, save it for later, because that's when the real conceptual development can occur.

The roles now become active and passive. Whoever becomes the giver would have been designated the job of

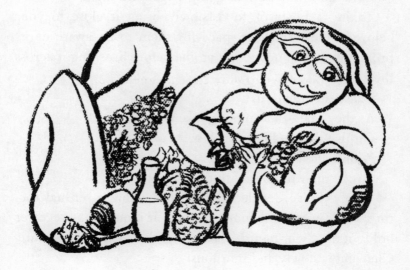

preparing a number of 'special' treats that the partner who is receiving does not know about.

After you've gone through the ceremony of entering your sanctuary, disrobing each other and initiating intimacy, whoever is the receiver should be lying on their back with their eyes closed.

The ideal erotic dessert is totally open to suggestion and is only limited by the extent of your imagination. Mangoes, lychees, custard apples, grapes, creamy desserts such as mousse, tiramisu, cream cake, ice-cream, sticky puddings, condiments like honey, chocolate or caramel sauce and of course maple syrup!

With your beloved settled, slowly relax them by softly stroking their body and face and lightly kissing them. They should breathe deeply, being aware of all the sensations going on around them.

> 'A GOOD COOK IS LIKE A
> SORCERESS WHO DISPENSES
> HAPPINESS.'
>   Elsa Schiaparelli

Taking a piece of food, slowly bring it close to your beloved's mouth. Allow space for them to be aware of its proximity and to inhale the aroma before brushing it across their lips.

Tease them with it.

As they open their mouth, take it away.

Or give them a big, juicy kiss.

Nibble their ears.

Stroke their nipples with the piece of food.

When you've decided they've had enough sensual torture, you can ease the morsel into their mouth. The receiver holds it in their mouth, savouring the taste and texture. Chewing it slowly and sensuously.

Being the giver, you may like to join in by placing a piece of food in your mouth and passing it to your lover through a kiss. As you allow the food to move from mouth to mouth, slowly letting it melt, the experience is likely to be elevated to a mutually erotic encounter.

What you will begin to discover is that by sharing food in this manner you will experience a merging of your two entities. The duality becoming a single persona brought into an orgasmic state by a single piece of food.

As the desire becomes intensified, the blindfold can be removed and the roles reversed.

By this time the subtle formality of a blindfold is probably not necessary and what you do with the food is up to you.

With the roles reversed, giver and receiver will continue to interconnect as you feed each other.

You can rub food all over each other's bodies and eat it off.

You can pour it over each other and lick it off.

You can take a mouthful of juice or champagne and share it with the other in a passionate kiss.

When it comes to food and sex, there are no rules.

Let your imagination loose!

Unleash your creative spirit!

Bon appétit.

'APPETITE GROWS
WITH EATING.'
French proverb

BECOMING
THE DANCE

> 'WILL YOU, WON'T YOU,
> WILL YOU, WON'T YOU,
> WILL YOU JOIN THE DANCE?'
> Lewis Carroll

WE, as human beings, were born to dance.

To move and sway to a particular rhythm, letting our energy and emotions take hold.

Dancing is an intrinsic component of sex.

For in the dance, we are able to let go of our inhibitions and allow our sense of freedom to express whatever it is we are feeling.

Whether it is the wild, abandoned movement of high voltage rock and roll or the tight togetherness of slow dancing in the big city, it is dance that conveys and elevates our sexual energy.

Dancing need not be limited to those odd occasions when you may be at a party or club but can become a regular part of your everyday life.

Dancing is especially energising in the morning, to get the heart started and to awaken the mind and spirit.

Or in the late afternoon, to shake off the rigours of a hard day's work and to boost energy levels.

What is stopping you, right now, putting your favourite dance track on and letting go in your living room or office? It doesn't matter what time of the day it is or whether you are alone or with someone.

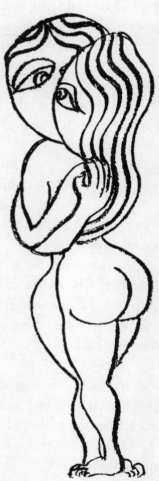

When you dance, feel the way your body pulsates.

Feel how it connects you to your power.

Feel the freedom.

Move your hips and pelvis in time with the music.

Lift your chest and arms and shake your head.

Exaggerate your movements.

Keep breathing, deep down into your belly.

And be aware of the exhalation. The letting go of the tension, fears and inhibitions.

Don't stop at just one track.

See if you can keep dancing for half an hour or more.

Use the whole room.

Make noise by yelling and hollering.

You will be amazed at how alive you'll begin to feel.

Dancing can also be soft and sensuous, especially when you are with your partner.

Play a slow song and hold your beloved really close so that your bodies – the entire length – are touching.

Put your arms around each other and move your hips together, slowly, in time with the beat.

Let your faces touch.

Cheek to cheek.

Let your hands run through each other's hair.

And down their back and buttocks.

Allow a synchronicity to develop between you.

Breathe in your beloved's aroma.

Lightly kiss their neck.

Their ears.

Their nose.

Their mouth.

Surrender yourself to the passion.

The desire.

Keeping your body moving.

Close your eyes and drown yourself in the music, the movement and the sensation.

In the highly likely event that you become aroused, don't be embarrassed, just stay with the dance, be with your lover, keep breathing … and surrender.

You are the dance and the dance is you.

As you go through life, may your dance card always be full.

> 'WE OUGHT DANCE WITH
> RAPTURE THAT WE SHOULD
> BE ALIVE AND IN THE FLESH
> AND PART OF THE LIVING
> INCARNATE COSMOS.'
>
> D. H. Lawrence

THE ESSENCE
OF POETRY

In its purity and softness, poetry is the most powerful of emotional forces.

For poetry is the expression of emotion.

An important source from which we recognise and honour the beauty of the other.

An outlet that reveals the reality of our passion.

A gathering of our collective thoughts.

Thoughts that delve deep into the conscious.

And unconscious.

In poetry you can say what you feel.

And feel what you say.

And feeling is that unique element that makes poetry poetic.

Much of this book is written in poetic form.

Because in many ways poetry is a fundamental way in which we can express intimacy and sensuality.

But the real beauty of poetry is that you don't have to be a poet to write it.

'GENUINE POETRY CAN COMMUNICATE BEFORE IT IS UNDERSTOOD.'
T. S. Eliot

And within us all is the gift of poetry.

Short lines.

Long thoughts.

With no need to rhyme or even make sense. Just the outflow of feelings that can run from one verse to many pages.

You may well ask 'What has poetry got to do with sex?'

The answer is it has everything to do with sex.

Because, in poetry, you are allowing your sensual, intimate nature to spring forth and be heard.

To say those things you wouldn't or couldn't ordinarily say.

The secret to writing a poem is to allow your thoughts to flow in a random manner.

To think about the person to whom you wish to express love, then write down the first thing that comes into your head.

And not to stop writing.

All you have to remember is to keep your sentences short.

If it sounds like gibberish, don't worry.

Some of the most beautiful poetry ever written is gibberish.

Allow your feelings about your beloved to run out of your mind and into your pen.

Eventually, you will come to an end, just as you found a beginning.

The final result may well surprise you. As it will your beloved.

In fact, one of the most inspiring ways to write poetry is together.

Sitting in your special space, each take a pad and pen and start expounding your inner emotions.

Giving yourselves no longer than ten or fifteen minutes.

If anything, poetry is spontaneous.

When you have finished, read your poems to each other.

Read them with warmth and tenderness.

Read them glancing into the other's eyes.

Read them observing the reflection of each other's sensitivity.

As well as this, be aware of any emotional change that takes place inside yourself and how you feel as both the giver and receiver.

Because poetry comes straight from the heart, it is one of the most precious gifts you can bestow upon your beloved.

> 'LOVE IS THE POETRY OF THE SENSES.'
> Honoré de Balzac

THESE three little words.
What do they really mean?
The admission of a feeling?
The confirmation of a relationship?
The ultimate expression of truth?
Or maybe a projection of
one's own inner need?
In a close and
connected
relationship
there will
always be
love. How
this love is
manifested
is a different
matter. For
when we are
with our partner, we
feel an overwhelming
sense of pleasure, security and well-being.

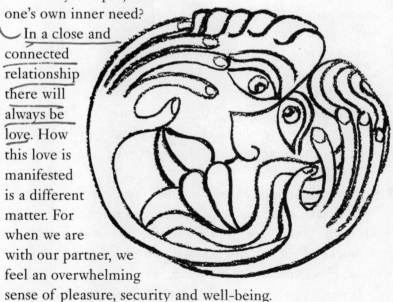

A force encompasses our body and a sense of euphoria clouds our mind.

This could be described as being a feeling of love.

But it is not necessarily love without.

It is also love within.

For love is an individual experience and in consequence of this, it must remain so.

Therefore, the utterance to another that you love them may not express what you're really feeling. Nor is love necessarily what the other person is feeling.

In essence, saying 'I love you' creates an obligation on the other. In other contexts it may be just an easy way out of a difficult situation. This can be the case regardless of whether the other person reciprocates the sentiment.

What you are really articulating at this point, is that when you are with your beloved, and for that matter, when you aren't with them, you feel a great deal of love within yourself.

> 'AN OUNCE OF LOVE IS WORTH A POUND OF KNOWLEDGE.'
> John Wesley

For this is the truth.

The feeling of love and the passing on of that feeling.

How deep are the feelings you have when you are together with your beloved? How genuine is the love?

Sit facing your beloved, looking into their eyes.

Each take it in turns to be speaker and listener. When one talks, the other maintains eye contact and makes no comment. What you are going to tell your beloved is all of those things you love about them.

For this process to really have meaning, you have to be absolutely open and honest with each other.

Say whatever comes into your head, no matter how trivial it seems. This goes beyond the process discussed in the chapter 'The alchemy of honesty'. For this is the unlocking of your feelings surrounding passion and intimacy.

For the man, you may love her freckles, her nose, the way she cooks lasagne, the way she puts on her stockings, the way she licks your ears, her imagination, her spirit and so on.

For the woman, you may love his smile, his teeth, the way he cooks lasagne, his underwear, his taste in shirts, the way he strokes your back, his humour, his spontaneity …

As you'll discover, the love you express to your partner unlocks the love you feel about yourself.

Love is life's most powerful energy and when you are being intimate with your beloved, it is this energy that forms the connection between you.

The energy that allows 'I love you' to transcend being a throw-away line.

Because on this level the sharing of sentiments of love between partners constitutes the very highest level of unity.

It is at this point – when each of you feel your love through the force of your togetherness – that it will feel right to look into your beloved's eyes and whisper 'I love you'.

And this is something that is all-pervasive.

This is something that is divine.

This is the true manifestation of love.

OVERCOMING
A HEADACHE

ONE of the barriers that stands in the way of achieving intimacy is the lack of the perfect environment.

Or the perfect mood.

Or the perfect partner.

So we compensate for our situation by coming up with the perfect rationalisation.

'I've got a headache.'

'I'm not feeling well.'

'My back hurts.'

'I'm tired.'

A multiplicity of excuses.

Objections that come out of fear.

That contribute to a lack of motivation.

Which results in denial.

For what you are denying is the best cure of all to ease these problems.

Sex is as regenerative as it is relaxing.

> 'WHEN THE HEAD ACHES, ALL THE BODY IS OUT OF TUNE.'
> Cervantes

> 'GRUMBLING IS THE DEATH OF LOVE.'
> Marlene Dietrich

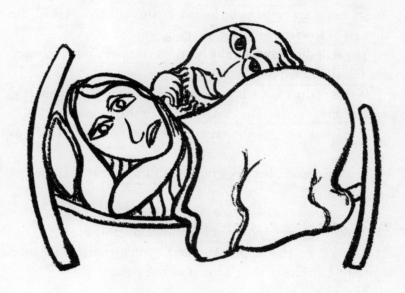

If you're feeling lethargic, it will boost your energy.
If you're suffering from insomnia, it will help you sleep.
If you're feeling ravenous, it will satisfy your hunger.

And as you've already read in this book, sex need not get physical. For being one with the other is all you need to achieve intimacy.

Even so, it seems we are forever creating barriers in our search for this intimacy.

Barriers that are often so well hidden that they only surface when we are confronted by something new, something out of the ordinary or something that is beyond our realm of experience.

And these barriers only exist because of a lack of communication and honesty between people.

Once you start sharing your fears and apprehensions about intimacy with your beloved you will have taken the first steps towards breaking them down.

You will discover that the barriers you put up to intimacy are usually based on a past experience.

If this is the case, what you need to remember is that sex, as with life, needs to be experienced in the moment.

The past no longer exists and the future has yet to happen.

It is this point, between past and future, that is known as eternity.

And eternity is the place where you are right now.

A place where no barrier is insurmountable.

As long as you approach this moment with a positive attitude, barriers will be a thing of the past.

And so too will headaches.

> 'ANXIETY IS LOVE'S GREATEST KILLER, BECAUSE IT IS LIKE THE STRANGE HOLD OF DROWNING.'
> Anais Nin

JUST how much we expect from each other is an interesting aspect of our relationships.

We look to our partner to be not only our lover, but also our confidant, nurturer, comrade, supporter, buddy, provider, and soul mate.

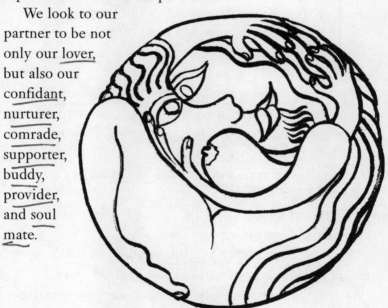

Our expectations go beyond what we want from our partner to the anticipation of how they feel or act or understand.

When it comes to our feelings we all have different methods with which we convey our expectations. However, to assume blithely what our partner anticipates is to be ignorant of the other person's individuality.

High expectations are usually the result of poor communication, resulting in many an erotic liaison wilting under the pressure of unsatisfied desires.

> 'WHEN LOVELY WOMAN STOOPS TO FOLLY
> AND FINDS TOO LATE THAT MEN BETRAY
> WHAT CHARM CAN SOOTH HER MELANCHOLY,
> WHAT ART CAN WASH HER GUILT AWAY?'
>
> Oliver Goldsmith

This pressure is our neediness getting out of control.

And, in our quest for gratification, unwittingly or unknowingly our expectations manifest themselves as demands.

Demands we put on our partners and ourselves.

We demand comfort.

We demand loving.

We demand attention.

This search invariably leads to conflict, as much of the pressure originates from our own self-centred space.

We believe that to satisfy our neediness we must seek satisfaction at whatever cost. This may well cover any number of criteria ranging from the pressure to perform to the pressure to do things against one's will.

By meeting a demand, you are creating a precedent.

By having a demand accepted you have won a false victory.

What this means is that in order to keep the peace, either together or individually, you have decided to either compromise a situation or be somebody you are not.

Neither of these scenarios will work, as they mean you have given away something of yourself.

Succumb to a demand and you are both selling yourselves short.

Pressure also comes in the form of possessiveness and jealousy. Those feelings that happen within us when we distrust or are envious of our partner. When we see them doing something we can't do, when they leave us out of a part of their life, or when we see them talking or flirting with another person.

Jealousy is the most destructive of emotions because it often results in irrational actions. We not only get mad, but also seek to get even.

Get even? For what?

Jealousy is not the responsibility of the other person, it is the responsibility of you.

Jealousy, as well as neediness, expectation and all the other projections we create in our relationships, is a product of the ego. It is the ego that stands in the way of most people's search for true happiness.

> 'MANIFEST PLAINNESS,
> EMBRACE SIMPLICITY,
> REDUCE SELFISHNESS,
> HAVE FEW DESIRES.'
>
> Lao-Tzu

By eliminating the ego, you can eliminate any need to create pressure.

By remaining centred and loving, you will discover that life has an ebb and flow of its own.

That there is no need to demand what it is you think you need.

Especially from your partner.

Solutions are found as long as you communicate to each other what it is you really want.

And in any loving and mutually compassionate relationship, most needs, wants and desires are easily satisfied.

In the expression of sensuality and intimacy, the real thrill is to expect the unexpected.

Allowing you and your beloved to be whatever it is you are and, in so doing, eliminating disappointment, rejection and bitterness.

If there is no expectation, then there is no demand.

It will either be, or not be.

And if it is to be, allow all those things you want to come into your life without the need to go searching for them.

If things are meant to happen to you, they will.

Give to yourself and they will give to you.

> 'LET THERE BE SPACES IN
> YOUR TOGETHERNESS.'
>   Kahlil Gibran

TURNING OUT
THE LIGHTS

To see or not to see.

To look or not to look.

We are a visual world.

We observe, analyse, scrutinise and form opinions on what our eyes see.

Yet what it is we see is often not the truth. For when you take in all the other senses, sight is only a very small part.

> 'WHEN THE LIGHT IS THERE, THE DARKNESS DISAPPEARS ... DARKNESS DOES NOT EXIST AT ALL, IT IS ONLY AN ABSENCE OF LIGHT.'
>
> Osho Rajneesh

And a very intangible part at that.

For in sight, we see only image, not substance.

It is touch, sound, smell and taste that add dimension.

We tend, too easily, to evaluate another person from a purely visual aspect.

However, being intimate in the dark can only happen once you are comfortable together in the light.

And not the other way around.

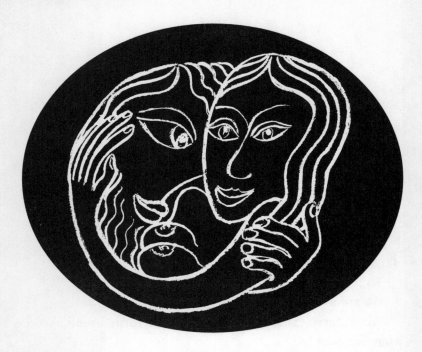

If you feel a need to turn the lights out because you are fearful of seeing and being seen, then you will need to work through the 'loving yourself' exercises earlier in this book.

Being with each other with the light off, or better still while one or both of you is blindfolded, can add to the erotic experience by enhancing all the other senses.

For as you touch, lick, fondle and embrace each other, a new twist in the sensual nature of your encounter comes into play.

The sound of each other's breathing.

The smell of the other's skin.

The taste of each other's juices.

The feeling as your hands touch and caress those warm and delicious parts of each other.

The darkness will lend itself to a build-up in intensity that creates its own unique kind of energy.

The more open and free you are about your intimacy, the more pleasurable will be the darkness.

For in the darkness you will see more of each other than you ever thought possible.

Lights out?

> 'DARKNESS IS MORE
> PRODUCTIVE OF SUBLIME
> IDEAS THAN LIGHT.'
> Edmund Burke

THE MOVEMENT
OF ENERGY

IN Western societies we tend to perceive our bodies and our beings on a purely physical and mental level.

Whereas much of Eastern philosophy teaches us that we are nothing more than <u>interconnected layers</u> of energy.

This energy not only circulates throughout our physical bodies, but also around us as an <u>aura</u> or <u>energy field</u>.

A practical illustration of how you generate ener-

> 'LIFE BEGETS LIFE. ENERGY CREATES ENERGY. IT IS BY SPENDING ONESELF THAT ONE BECOMES RICH.'
> Sarah Bernhardt

gy is best exemplified when you become aware of such instinctive feelings as <u>intuition or premonition</u>. Consider the way your mood may alter when a person enters your space, either invited or uninvited.

Do your muscles tense or relax?

Do you get a nervous pain in the pit of your stomach?

Do you tend to change colour or perspire?

These sensations are nothing more than the <u>transferring and intermingling</u> of energy.

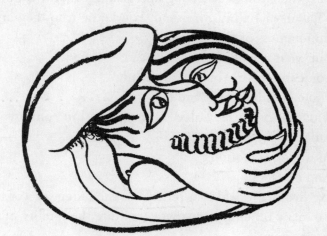

It is this energy that is linked to our internal rhythm.

Our heartbeat.

Our pulse.

The continuous vibration that resonates throughout our bodies every second, every minute, every hour, every day, every week, every month and every year of our lives.

Each of us has a unique rhythmic signature that creates its own energy field.

It is this collection of substance that makes the individual within us an exceptional human being.

When we talk of individuality, we need to understand that this means every person on this planet has a different face.

A different fingerprint.

A different voice pattern.

When you answer the phone and a familiar voice is on the other end, you know who it is without even seeing their face.

Just as when you hear a song being sung by Phil Collins or Bob Dylan or Barbra Streisand. You know who they are by the uniqueness of their voice.

But what is voice?

You can't see it. You can't touch it.

You can only hear it and feel it.

This is because voice is nothing but energy and vibrations.

As are our emotions.

And our feelings.

We live in a world that relies on visual identity, yet there are so many other aspects that constitute the totality of who we are as people.

When you become entwined with your lover, what you are creating is pure energy.

The energy that happens when individuals connect.

> 'FOR PASSION HAS COME TO THE VERGE AND LEAPS,
> HEADLONG TO THE BLIND ABYSS,
> YET GATHERS THEREBY THE STRENGTH OF DEEPS,
> AND EDDIES A MOMENT AND SWIRLS AND SWEEPS,
> TILL PERIL IS ONE WITH BLISS.'
>
> Harriet L. Childe-Pemberton

It is this connection that creates new energy fields that are virtually electric and are greater than, yet different from, the sum of their parts.

When next you are with your beloved, be aware of the way you feel when you are close to them.

Do they turn you on just by their presence?

Do you feel weak or strong?

Do you feel desired or rejected?

Do you feel connected?

It is the way you interact energetically that is the secret behind all successful relationships.

As you immerse yourself in the intensity of your fusion, you become lost in the realm of the ethereal. Bonded by a force that transcends the physical. By allowing your duality to merge into one entity, you will set forth an outflow of pulsations that resonate to a new beat.

You will discover that there is no necessity for physical contact.

That you can connect by looking into each other's eyes across a crowded room.

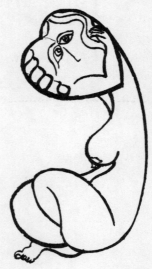

That you're always together, even when you're miles apart.

It is this atmosphere of spirituality that others around you will be drawn to.

You will witness in your togetherness the positive and lasting effect your combined radiance has on others.

The realisation that you are, and are surrounded by, an intangible and yet real totality.

To discover the infinite satisfaction that is possible on all levels.

Simply because we possess the ability to tap a source of internal power that transcends the physical act, giving sex a new significance.

The more powerful the energetic connection, the higher the ecstatic experience.

It is this that constitutes the true ethos that is an integral component of sex beyond intercourse.

> 'SEX IS ONE OF THE NINE
> REASONS FOR REINCARNATION.
> THE OTHER EIGHT AREN'T
> IMPORTANT.'
>
> Henry Miller

EJACULATION ...

... AS distinct from orgasm.

Because it is over rather quickly, ejaculation doesn't really allow a full body orgasm to occur.

Therefore, ejaculation should not be regarded as orgasm.

The old Chinese philosophers, who are reputed to have known about these things, described ejaculation as dropping your seed on the ground. This evaluation does have a ring of truth about it.

They also say that withholding ejaculation allows you to retain your sexual energy, giving you a renewed sense of vitality and vibrancy.

This is also true.

Another particular concern of men is penis size. As many women don't consider penis size to be important, there is no reason why it should worry men.

> 'GO TO BED WITH THE LAMB, AND RISE WITH THE LARK.'
>
> English proverb

The reality is that when it comes to making love, penis size is of little importance.

As we have discovered, a man need not even use his penis when making love.

Moreover, he can not only have an orgasm without ejaculating, he can have an orgasm without an erection.

In the desire to prolong a sexual encounter, it is important to note that the woman's orgasm is her own responsibility. While withholding ejaculation can be a factor in extending her experience, its primary objective is to enhance the man's pleasure, rather than the woman's.

Consequently, for a man to have a fuller, more meaningful orgasm, he should explore the exhilaration that can come with refraining from ejaculation.

Naturally, not having intercourse makes this easier, but even when a couple are being intimate, ejaculation can happen at any time.

The best way to avoid ejaculation, when you feel it coming on, is to stop what you are doing and start breathing deeply, drawing the breath in and out through your PC muscle.

Do not be afraid to communicate with your partner. (For the woman, when your beloved tells you to 'hold on', respect his wish, because you will want not only to share the moment but also to intensify it.)

When you do slow down, remember to keep breathing; as you do, concentrate on your genitals and the gradual subsiding of the feeling. At the same time you will experience a warm glow around the area. This is the subtle transferring of energy and the first stage of a total body orgasm.

The more times you stop and allow the feeling of ejaculation to pass, the more your orgasmic sensations will be internalised.

You may start to feel a vibration throughout your body. Try not to suppress this. Instead, on the outgoing breath, allow your body to relax. The shaking will just happen and as it does, it will create an extraordinary feeling.

With a little practice you will find the need to ejaculate becomes less frequent as the connection with your beloved deepens. You will also discover a lingering pleasure in your intimacy, with ejaculation no longer being an end in itself.

Not that you should totally force yourself to eliminate ejaculation altogether. Every now and again you may feel a real desire to let go and when this happens the ensuing release will be literally explosive. What you will now find is that you are more in control of the when and the how.

The build-up in sexual energy that is the result of non-ejaculation will not only heighten your overall pleasure but will make you, as a man, more aware of your orgasmic potential.

And hers.

ORGASM:
RIDING THE WAVE

O<small>H</small> yes.
 Yes!
 YES!
 <u>Orgasm is one of life's great affirmations.</u>
 It is the <u>state of mindlessness when your entire being</u>
<u>becomes totally ethereal.</u>

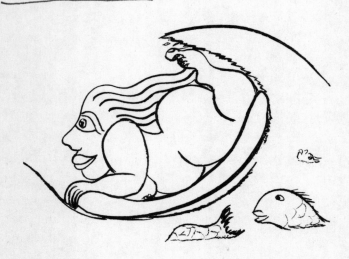

It is when time stands still.

The French call it *le petit mort,* the little death, for in many ways this is what happens when you are in orgasm.

You are in your body and out of your body.

In fact, you are more than your body.

You are pure energy.

Pure bliss.

Orgasm need not be localised, but can encompass your whole body.

Orgasm can come at any time, not just during intercourse.

It can occur while you are stroking.

Or massaging.

Or kissing.

Or even sitting together making eye contact.

The more you are in tune with yourself and, in turn, connected with your beloved, the more orgasmic you'll become.

And this is true for both the man and the woman.

One of the beauties of sex beyond intercourse is that it takes the pressure off the man to perform.

Orgasm is like riding a wave.

It comes on through the subtle shifting of energy.

Like ripples through your body.

Start breathing into these sensations as they take hold, usually in the area of the genitals or lower belly. Drawing the breath up through the PC muscle so that it merges with the orgasmic sensation.

For a man, this will not only assist you in controlling your ejaculation, but will allow you to experience the orgasmic sensation throughout your body.

During this process you must relax, allowing the energy to move you.

And it will.

All you have to do is place your trust in your higher self.

When you do, you'll find that your body will virtually take over. Your breathing will increase its rapidity and your mind will become empty.

The more you allow the feeling to flow, the more intense it will become.

Just surrender to whatever is happening.

And maintain your breathing.

Be aware of what's going on inside your body without trying to control it.

If you are embracing your partner, you will soon discover that your energies will become intertwined.

You will feel a part of each other.

Inside each other.

You will become encircled by an invisible bond. An energy field that draws you together.

So that you become one.

In harmonious splendour.

A state of abandon that may last five minutes, or if you allow it, almost indefinitely.

Don't fight it.

Ecstasy is good for you.

INTERCOURSE
AND BEYOND ...

IT may appear that the philosophy behind this book is that one should avoid intercourse.

Far from it.

What this book seeks to point out is the fact that intercourse alone does not constitute the totality of sex.

The act of intercourse has been discussed to such an extent that most people tend to regard it as a kind of sexual focal point.

It isn't.

> 'FREEDOM FROM THE DESIRE FOR AN ANSWER IS ESSENTIAL TO UNDERSTANDING THE PROBLEM.'
>
> J. Krishnamurti

As you may have discovered in these pages, there is an amazing variety of choices when it comes to exploring and sharing your sexuality, of which intercourse is but one aspect. Albeit one of a certain importance.

If the activity you are involved in leads to the desire for genital penetration, then let it happen with that same spirit of connectedness as the rest of your lovemaking, rather than by forcing the issue.

When it comes to intercourse there is much conjecture about which position is best. There is no shortage of books that go into graphic detail on the multiplicity of ways in which a man can insert his penis into his beloved's vagina. According to the Kamasutra, there are sixty-four ways … and then some more. However, most people who are loving and open about their sexuality tend to discover which positions are most comfortable for them without the need of a manual. These days it seems that too much importance is placed on the gymnastic variations one must attempt in order to gain sexual satisfaction.

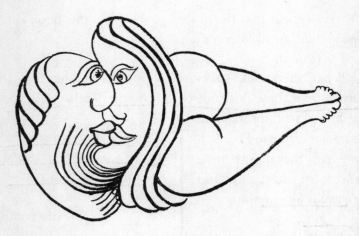

For you to be able to maintain your energetic and spiritual connection, the most satisfying positions will generally be face to face (either man or woman on top), seated (woman on man's lap) or lying side by side. Being in this union will allow you to synchronise your breathing and to kiss and caress each other and maintain eye contact, all of which make up the key components of the overall act of making love.

Let your bodies unite, becoming one with the other, not only by physical connection, but also by a merging of your two energies. For within your orgasmic duality, no matter which position you have intercourse in, you and your beloved will still become one entity, locked together in mutual ecstasy.

As already discussed, the crucial element in prolonging the act is for the man to withhold ejaculation.

For the man, if the anxiety to ejaculate is too powerful then by all means let it go. Withholding ejaculation does not mean holding it in when the feeling becomes too uncomfortable. You should be at ease with your orgasm and, in time, you will discover the joy of channelling your orgasmic energy throughout your body. This applies both for the man and the woman.

Men will find, with a little practice, that the need to ejaculate will begin to subside, but the resultant stillness will start to generate another energy. This is known as the valley orgasm — that for both of you will start in stillness rather than evolving out of activity.

The valley orgasm begins like a surge of pleasure throughout your bodies, as you both start to vibrate. When this happens, keep breathing together, simultaneously or alternately (as in the circular breathing exercise explained in the chapter 'The breath of life'). As one of you exhales, the other inhales. The man draws the energy in through the heart and out through the penis, while the woman draws the breath in through the vagina and out through the heart. This way of sharing the breath, once mastered, has the ability to take you to a higher plateau.

As you let go into the union, remember to stay present in the moment by not closing your eyes, as when they are closed they take you away from where you are. For some people, opening the eyes during intercourse may take some getting used to. However, by starting with a few seconds at a time, you will slowly work your way up to where you are able to keep your eyes open naturally. This will allow you to look at your partner during intercourse, giving you a deeper and much more loving perspective as you watch the change that occurs in your beloved's face, seeing the love in their eyes, being a part of their ecstasy.

And intercourse is more than putting your head down and just 'going for it'. You can still continue to do many of those other things described in this book such as kissing, stroking, biting, scratching, licking, whispering, screaming or whatever.

Conversely, you may desire to take a soft and sensual approach, allowing your liaison to flow languidly like a river.

Whichever way it happens, you will eventually feel the heat of energy build up, until you reach that point where you lose yourself in a wave of high-voltage orgasmic bliss.

As this happens, surrender into it, as the way to extend the encounter is to stay in your body and that of your beloved.

The ultimate outcome of love is not sex.

It is meditation.

And when sex, especially intercourse, transcends to a meditative level, then it becomes an ecstatic experience.

Hallelujah!

... AND BEYOND

THE question may have crossed your mind 'Would oral sex constitute sex beyond intercourse?'

The answer is yes.

That being said, oral sex is a practice that is regarded by many as the ultimate taboo, because the juices that flow during oral sex are confused with those passed during elimination.

As such, oral sex is incorrectly perceived as being dirty. This assumption is basically incorrect provided you have bathed near the time of making love.

As your relationship with your beloved expands, you will find many of the exercises in this book leading you to kissing, stroking and licking each other's genitals.

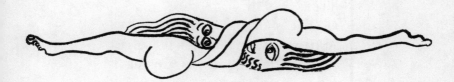

From this perspective, savouring and tasting each other's vital essences is intimacy at its most profound.

The act of mouth-to-genital contact between you and your beloved becomes one of the deepest expressions of your love.

What makes oral sex such an ecstatic experience is that, in a way, it takes us back to our early years, to the time of our birth.

For a man to give to a woman is, symbolically, a return to the womb. For a woman to give to a man is to revert to the role of being breast fed.

The key to oral sex is communication, to treat your beloved gently and to set your boundaries. However, gaining the most out of oral sex involves a certain degree of risk.

'I AM A TRUE ADORER OF LIFE AND IF I CAN'T REACH THE FACE OF IT I PLANT MY KISS SOMEWHERE LOWER DOWN.'

Saul Bellow

The more risk you take, the more beautiful the experience.

Because oral sex opens up a world of ecstatic possibilities.

The deeper you go, the more you will discover.

Thus oral sex will become the most potent test of your trust for each other.

'I LET DOWN MY SILKEN HAIR,
OVER MY SHOULDERS,
AND OPEN MY THIGHS OVER MY LOVER,
"TELL ME, IS THERE ANY PART OF ME
THAT IS NOT LOVEABLE".'

Tzu Yeh

MAKING IT FUN

IN recent times, many aspects about our sexuality have become deadly serious.

There is the spectre of AIDS and the various other sexually related afflictions.

There is the concern between partners about performance, intimacy and ultimate satisfaction.

There is the problem individuals have in dealing with their aloneness.

There is the guilt and shame inherent within many of us, when our belief systems are challenged, invaded or brought into question.

'TO FEAR LOVE, IS TO FEAR LIFE AND THOSE WHO FEAR LIFE ARE ALREADY THREE PARTS DEAD ... TO CONQUER FEAR IS THE BEGINNING OF WISDOM.'
Bertrand Russell

There is the fear to confront our problems and seek solutions.

With all of this going on, is it any wonder that for many, the real joy has gone out of sex?

Because those things you believed about sex were really difficult to achieve.

And, for you, sex has no intimacy.

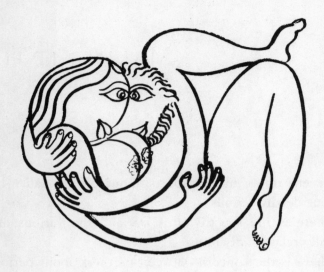

Are these the reasons you have read this book?

You will have discovered by now a lot about intimacy and sensuality and the relationship they have to the way you are as a sexual being.

But, if I am to advocate any single thing about sex, it is, first and foremost, fun.

By fun, I mean treating sex in a light-hearted way.

Viewing sex as the happy, playful and exuberant pursuit it really is.

All the exercises and suggestions you have read about in this book have to be done in the spirit of fun. While you will have moments of sadness, anger and catharsis, these should all be compensated by giving equal time to laughter and being joyful.

Start by making your beloved laugh.

Tickle them where you know they're ticklish.
Lick them where you know they're sensitive.
Bite them where you know they're vulnerable.
If, in the heat of passion you want to break out giggling …
Giggle.
Share the joke.
Be joyful in the merriment.
It won't affect your performance.
Rather, it will break down a lot of barriers.
Fun in sex exemplifies the fact that two people are more than just lovers.
They are friends.
And friends play with each other.
Because playing is fun.
This is the true essence of this thing called sex.

> 'A DESIRE TO HAVE ALL THE
> FUN IS NINE-TENTHS OF THE
> LAW OF CHIVALRY.'
>   Dorothy L. Sayers

BITS AND PIECES

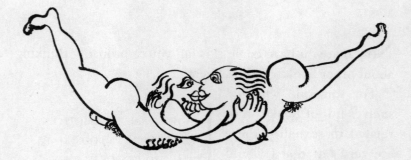

FURTHER READING

Now that you have come this far, you're probably thinking about other books on the subject.

For someone who has shelves full of books on or related to sexuality, there are very few that I would recommend. This is not because they aren't worthwhile, it is because they will only serve to confuse.

> 'THERE ARE TWO MOTIVES FOR READING A BOOK; ONE, THAT YOU ENJOY IT, THE OTHER, THAT YOU CAN BOAST ABOUT IT.'
>
> Bertrand Russell

As already mentioned, many books on sex talk about the physicality without the intimacy. In fact the word 'intimacy' is rarely discussed in most conventional books that deal with the subject of sex.

Because I take a somewhat spiritual approach to sexuality, I would suggest that those of you curious enough to want to delve a little deeper should look for books that deal with the subject from this perspective.

Six of the best are:

- *The Art of Sexual Ecstasy*, Margot Anand (The Aquarian Press)

- *Sexual Secrets*, Nik Douglas and Penny Slinger (Destiny Books)
- *Sacred Sexuality*, Georg Feuerstein (Tarcher/Perigee)
- *Passions of Innocence*, Stuart Sovatsky (Destiny Books)
- *The Encyclopedia of Erotic Wisdom*, Rufus C. Camphausen (Inner Traditions International)
- *The End of Sex*, George Leonard (Bantam)

Happy reading!

MUSIC:
THE FOOD OF LOVE

WHAT makes music the food of love may well be in the listening. Or in the context of *This thing called sex*, not listening.

If you utilise music as part of your lovemaking you should take care that what you play enhances the ambience rather than overpowers it.

I recall a radio station asking its listeners to phone in with their favourite 'bonking' songs. The suggestions ranged from the sublime to the outrageous.

Whether you like to make love to Pearl Jam or Pavarotti, the right kind of music is a purely subjective decision.

You may find that a particular music track, especially one that is a favourite, will have the effect of taking you away from the space where you are. In this context heavy rock, opera, techno or country music will tend to make strange bedfellows.

The type of music that works best in an intimate situation will have a more mystical, almost hypnotic quality about it. What this

> 'IN MUSIC THE PASSIONS ENJOY THEMSELVES ... WITHOUT MUSIC, LIFE WOULD BE A MISTAKE.'
> Friedrich Nietzsche

means is that the melodic structure has a way of integrating itself with the mood of the moment. In other words, it is not the type of music that will have you singing along.

There is an ever-increasing range of ambient and ethereal music, much of it extraordinarily beautiful. Most larger record stores carry a wide variety and they will generally allow you to listen before you buy.

Two other sources of this type of music are mail-order organisations: New World Productions, PO Box 244, Red Hill, Queensland, 4059 and MRA Entertainment Group, PO Box 703, Mount Gravatt, Queensland, 4122. They produce a regular catalogue in full colour with descriptions of all tracks and a money-back guarantee.

A list of titles follows (many available through New World). They are tried and trusted, not only from personal experience but also from requests made after workshops.

- *Spiritual Environment – Shamanic Dream*, Anugama (Nightingale)
- *Spiritual Environment – Tantra*, Anugama (Nightingale)
- *Excalibur*, Medwyn Goodall (New World)
- *Merlin*, Medwyn Goodall (New World)
- *Zen*, Terry Oldfield (New World)

- *1492 Conquest of Paradise*, Vangelis (EastWest)
- *MCMXC*, Enigma (Virgin)
- *The Cross of Changes*, Enigma (Virgin)
- *Atlantis Angelis*, Patrick Bernhardt (Imagine)
- *Solaris Universalis*, Patrick Bernhardt (Imagine)
- *Shamanyka*, Patrick Bernhardt (Imagine)
- *Beyond Recall*, Klaus Shulze (Venture)
- *The Mission*, Ennio Morricone (Virgin)
- *Passion*, Peter Gabriel (Real World)
- *Yamantaka,* Hart, Wolff and Hennings (Celestial Harmonies)

Note: Terry Oldfield, Vangelis, Steve Halpern and Medwyn Goodall have produced many titles, all of which are worth listening to along with most of the titles on the Nightingale label.

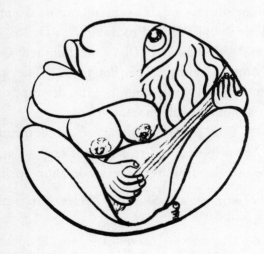

WHAT ...
NO INDEX?

IF you peruse the index of any number of books on the subject of sex you will discover that words such as *intimacy* or *sensuality* or even *love* rarely get a mention.

Not so in this book. These words are mentioned regularly.

So if you are looking for an index that will lead you to all the juicy bits, forget it.

This whole book is juicy.

And the way to get the most out of it is to start at the beginning.

Besides, the chapter headings will lead you to any specific subject you may be looking for.

Enjoy!

'THERE ARE THE MEN WHO PRETEND TO UNDERSTAND A BOOK BY SCOUTING THROUGH THE INDEX, AS IF A TRAVELLER SHOULD GO ABOUT DESCRIBING A PALACE WHEN HE HAD SEEN NOTHING BUT THE PRIVY.'

Jonathan Swift

Everything you wanted to know about the author but were afraid to ask

During the writing of this book, the most common question asked of me was whether it is based on experience.

The short answer is yes.

If it wasn't, I would not have been able to write it.

In the realm of running workshops (or playgroups, as I now call them) I have come to the realisation that unless one has been through the experience, it is nearly impossible to take others through it.

So what are the qualifications needed to write a book on sex?

The answer to this question is none. Because there are none.

One of America's leading psychotherapists, James Hillman, best summed it up in the title of a book he co-authored: *There's Been a Hundred Years of Psychotherapy and the World is Getting Worse.*

For those who may still be interested, I am an advertising copywriter by profession and have slowly weaned myself away from this one-dimensional world to a path that is somewhat more spiritual.

Coming to terms with the exploration of sexuality involves intuition, understanding and a great deal of awareness.

This is not to say that I haven't studied and practised various methods, processes and disciplines that have led me to the perception I now have of sex. I have. These include yoga, Tantra, breath therapy, meditation and massage.

My time is now taken up with writing and facilitating sexuality and relationship playgroups (see the next chapter). I also conduct corporate and community training programs around meditation, creativity and team-building.

As to whether or not I have tapped what is the essence of sex, then only the content of this book can answer that.

As Duke Ellington once said, 'If it sounds good, it is good.'

> 'THERE IS NO PSYCHOLOGY;
> THERE IS ONLY BIOGRAPHY
> AND AUTOBIOGRAPHY.'
> Thomas Szasz

FURTHER EXPLORATION

As you will no doubt realise by now, much of *This thing called sex* is based on the concept that sex is not an end in itself but an expression of love.

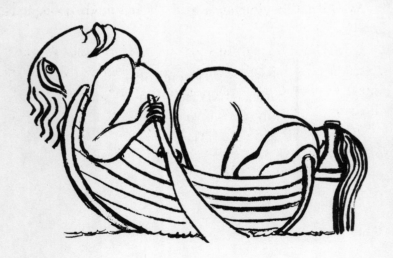

And the real way to discover and understand more about uplifting your sexuality and rediscovering love is not in the reading.

It is in the doing.

For this reason, I conduct an extensive program of group activities based on the precepts discussed in this book. I refer to these as playgroups rather than workshops.

The playgroup concept is designed to avoid the confrontationist aspect that is prevalent in many workshops that claim to deal with issues around relationships and sexuality. Each playgroup is non-threatening and presented in a space that is playful, nurturing and safe.

> 'WE ARE ASTONISHED AT THOUGHT, BUT SENSATION IS EQUALLY WONDERFUL.'
> Voltaire

Most importantly, they are conducted in an atmosphere of fun.

I facilitate playgroups on a regular basis in most Australian capital cities and regional centres. If you are interested in more information you can call, fax or write to the address below:

Sex Beyond Intercourse, Box 6478, St Kilda Road, Melbourne, Victoria, Australia, 3004

Phone: (03) 9820 2991

Fax: (03) 9820 2997

> 'IF WE GO ON EXPLAINING, WE
> SHALL CEASE TO UNDERSTAND
> ONE ANOTHER.'
>
> Talleyrand